ISBN 0-7414-3372-9

Published by:

INFINITY
PUBLISHING.COM

1094 New Dehaven Street, Suite 100
West Conshohocken, PA 19428-2713
Info@buybooksontheweb.com
www.buybooksontheweb.com
Toll-free (877) BUY BOOK
Local Phone (610) 941-9999
Fax (610) 941-9959

Printed in the United States of America

Printed on Recycled Paper

Published July 2006

KEEPING HEALTHY by KEEPING TRACK

Dedicated to our husbands Atul and Melvin,
and to our doctors: caretakers nonpareil.

ACKNOWLEDGMENTS

When it comes to personal health, absolutely everyone has a story, a drama, a successful stay in the hospital, a hideous mistake, a miracle, a reference to something just read or seen, a personal brush with tragedy, or a sure-fire remedy for whatever ails you. We are very grateful for all the many stories and tales of medical hits and misses.

We talked with dozens of people while working on this book. We listened and listened and learned as much from them as from our research.

Particular thanks are due to D'Arcy Webb, Katrina Streiff, M.D., Julie Noonan, Cynthia Heldt, M.D., Rich Jones, Jessica Rower, M.D., Melora Lucas, Annie Laurino, R.N., Amy Dwyer, Ingrid Lynch, Paul Seidenstat, PhD and Julia McNeil.

We also gleaned an enlightening amount of information from newspapers, magazines, television and the Internet, all of which are chock full of health news.

The generous professional advice, touching personal stories, extensive resources and continuing influx of information combined to convince us we were on the right track. It truly is important to have an easy and complete system for sorting it all out.

So thanks to all of you who contributed to our knowledge and helped us clarify and simplify.

Note: Although we have checked and double-checked the information contained in this book, we readily take responsibility for any errors.

CONTENTS

KEEPING HEALTHY by KEEPING TRACK

A Complete Guide to Maintaining Your Own Medical Records

This section contains charts providing background information and ongoing
monitoring of key aspects of your health. These charts are the foundation
of your record keeping system.

Emergency Information
Keeping an Ongoing Health Log
Appointments/Addresses
Current Health Profile and Significant Health History
Family Health History
Medications and Supplements
Labs and Tests

A LETTER TO OUR READERS

We all know how our bodies feel... sort of. We say, "I'm lucky. I'm pretty healthy I guess," and go our merry way. Or we might say, "I don't feel so hot today," and take an aspirin. Or we might just say, "Boy, I feel terrible!" and pick up the phone and call the doctor.

It's actually better to really know than to just guess. The only way to truly monitor the state of our health is to actually keep track of it, and this requires no more than a simple monitoring system.

In trying to get and stay healthy ourselves, we began to notice how many other people we know who are in the same boat. As Laura found herself waving a regretful goodbye to middle age, she searched out, and held onto for dear life, the treadmill at her nearest gym. As Lillian was dragged kicking and screaming into old age, she began to question her 30-year-old dieting system of "just don't pay any attention and it will all go away."

We realized we just might have to play a more active role in this "staying alive" business. We even began to think in terms of a full partnership with our doctors. (We both imagine their leafing through our thick, thick files and breathing a sigh of relief, "It's about time!")

We began to monitor our progress not just in our imagination but on paper. We realized over time that the clearer and simpler our systems, the easier it was to keep track, and the more success we had.

We aren't going to tell you what to do or how to do it. We are going to give you some basic information as well as some tools and guidelines for keeping track. We offer you everything we've learned while writing this book. Use any of our ideas you find helpful. Feel free to modify them or make up your own. If you come up with a quicker, easier way to record, be sure to let us know.

We're not doctors and we make no claims to having medical training of any kind. In this book we have included the best information we have been able to gather to date, and have listed key book and Internet resources.

Our format allows you to update your knowledge by keeping your eyes and ears open and by paying attention to newspapers, magazines, radio and TV news and the Internet. Most of all, you can gain solid information by listening to your doctors and by asking them to explain what you don't understand.

Keeping Healthy by Keeping Track is an effective personal health organizer. We offer it to you with our best wishes for a healthy, happy, and fun filled life.

Lillian Shah and Laura Messinger

P.S. Remember to keep it simple and consistent.

INTRODUCTION

WHAT IS GOOD HEALTH?

We Enjoy Good Health When We Are Sound in Mind, Body and Spirit.
The benefits of good health are well known. Good health brings energy, enthusiasm, enjoyment, good looks and longevity.

Being healthy is being:
- Disease free (or having chronic conditions under treatment and control).
- Physically fit and strong.
- Mentally alert and engaged.
- Emotionally happy and positive.
- Socially active and involved.
- Connected to self, spouse, family, friends, co-workers, community, and the world.

Healthy people know how important it is to their health to have a positive attitude and good self image. They are:
- Honest, fair, and trustworthy.
- Self-aware and realistic.
- Willing to do their fair share.
- Aware that joy is not an accident but a choice.
- Aware of their obligation to be socially attractive.
- Able to value others and avoid grumbling and criticizing.
- Tuned in and alert.
- Friendly.
- Welcome wherever they go.

Healthy people know drugs are dangerous and actively avoid drug abuse.
They know the danger of excessive use of alcohol; they avoid recreational drugs and they do not share or abuse prescription drugs.

Healthy people are prepared for sudden illness and inevitable decline.
They know their options and rights as health care consumers, and can make good decisions about:
- Health care systems
- Hospitals
- Follow-up options
- Health care providers
- Medications
- Insurance
- Tests and lab work
- Long term care

Proper Screenings
Healthy people know an ounce of prevention is worth a pound of cure. They are aware of and informed about the consequences of aging and normal wear and tear. Even when they are feeling fine and not at all stressed they:
- Get regular dental and physical checkups.
- Do routine medical screenings.
- Regularly monitor their weight, blood pressure, and heart beat.

Treatment
Healthy people form a partnership with their doctors. They listen to them and:
- Make appointments as needed.
- Follow recommended treatments.
- Give the doctor feedback if medication isn't working, or if unexpected side effects occur.
- Take their medications as prescribed.
- See specialists as advised.

WHY KEEP YOUR OWN MEDICAL RECORDS?

Why? **Because You Don't Just Want More — You Want Better**
It is a quality of life issue. After all, our goal is not just to live longer, but to stay well and to live better as we live longer. The responsibility for keeping track becomes yours because you will always be intimately involved in your own health care, whether you wish to be or not.

Why? **Because Record Keeping Answers the Basic Fact Questions**
As you accumulate your own personal medical information you will tend to keep in mind the questions: *who, what, when, where, how and why*? It's important to make sure you know the answers to every single one of them in every interaction with your doctors and health care practitioners, and all medical facilities.

Why? **Because They Affect You the Most**
You need to take charge of your own medical records and keep them in your own care. After all, who has more of a vested interest in your health than you, yourself? Who has more to gain from a healthier you?

Why? **For the Big Picture**
It's important to have ongoing awareness in order to prevent potential illnesses and avoid potential mistakes. To maintain good health practices and track our success, we must be aware of what we are *actually* doing as opposed to what we might *think* we are doing. It's particularly crucial to have accurate background information in case of a sudden health crisis.

Why? **So You Know**
It's important for you to be in possession of all information that pertains to you personally. The position of medical historian goes to you because you know the most about you and you care the most. You contain your own history, and are the most alert whenever significant references are made to you. You are most likely to take care that nothing important gets lost or misplaced. You will be the most diligent in charting your own progress from new or changed medication or from recommended lifestyle changes. You are the primary consultant when it comes to decision making in partnership with your doctor.

Why? **For Your Doctor**
   Too many patients: Most likely your doctor already has a lot of patients—as many as several hundred in most cases. In a group practice she might be in charge of several thousand additional patients when she is on call.

   Complicated Record Keeping: Your home records will be invaluable in case the doctor loses your records or can't access them for some reason.

   Errors: Because doctors and health practitioners do make mistakes, it's reassuring to know you can supply or validate any crucial information.

   Change of Doctor: If you change doctors due to the constraints of your insurance, or if something goes wrong in the transfer of records, your records will provide a solid backup.

   Second opinion: When seeking a second opinion, you can review your own records and make sure you understand and can articulate your concerns and questions.

***Why?* To Make Sure**
It's important to be especially vigilant when it comes to significant medical events. It's crucial to document dramatic medical events such as:

- Surgery
- Accidents, Injuries
- New Medications
- Evaluative Procedures
- Major Illnesses
- Emergencies
- Severe and Chronic Conditions

Always describe in detail: conditions, diagnoses, treatment, results and any complications. Constantly remind yourself that your records will be most informative and helpful when they answer the fact questions—*who, what, when, where, how and why.*

***Why?* In Case of Emergency**
Your records will be truly portable and easy to grab. In case of a disaster such as New Orleans, you could wind up in possession of the only copy of your medical information.

***Why?* To Avoid Costly or Deadly Mistakes**
98,000 people die each year from preventable medical errors such as operating on the wrong part of the body, giving the wrong medicine and delaying treatment. Most patients are generally aware that errors do occur in hospitals. It's important to know how they happen, and to know what one can do to help prevent them.

If you are informed and alert, you will be equipped to check each step of the way and make sure you are receiving the correct medication and the correct procedures. It is crucial to look out for the following possibilities because they do happen:

COMMON ERRORS

Handoffs: Many problems occur during handoffs. It's important to be especially vigilant when a patient is transferred to a different part of the hospital or from one health care person to another.

Misdiagnosis: Doctors today have busy schedules. They use numerous diagnostic tools and yet sometimes things are missed or incorrectly diagnosed. Be aware of the possibility of false positive or false negative test results, of X-rays reversed in view boxes, incompatible medications, or overlooked serious conditions which negatively affect each other.

Verbal errors: It's easy to misunderstand what is said aloud, especially when everyone is so busy. It should be, but it's not always the case, that staff members double check. Sometimes patients even receive treatment meant for another patient with a similar name. Without becoming a pest, ask for a repetition of any verbal directive you hear. Write it down if you can.

Lost, misplaced, inaccessible records: Look out for incomplete records in your file or records not being forwarded, received late, or lost. Even if they can find your records, it's difficult to get them from the hospital. A precise summary, however, is usually created when a patient leaves the hospital and is easy to transfer by fax, e-mail or regular mail. You have the right to this summary; remember to ask for it.

Mistakes involving surgery:
- Wrong surgical procedure
- Surgery on the wrong patient
- Surgery on the wrong body part
- Foreign objects left in the body after surgery

Carelessness:
- Careless checking of charts
- Lack of cleanliness resulting in staph infection

Bureaucracies, group practice, extensive reliance on tests and procedures, specialization, different types of record keeping, too many different people, too much paper—all add to the problem of medical mistakes.

AVOIDING MEDICAL MISTAKES

Ask questions: Speak up if you have concerns or don't understand what you are being told.

Take a helper: Get in the habit of taking a relative or friend along to help you.

Avoid a misdiagnosis: A diagnosis is made by considering numerous pieces of information. Most doctors are in a group practice and connected with a primary hospital so getting a second opinion or consulting with a colleague can be routine. Also, second opinions are paid for by most health insurance companies.

Know your medications: Keep a list of all the medicines you take and any drug allergies you may have. Tell your doctor about all the medicines you take, including over-the-counter medications, and herbs or supplements.

Get copies of all test results: Ask the doctor or nurse when and how you will get test results and ask what the results mean. Always try to get them immediately, at the time of the test, or at the time your doctor is reviewing them with you.

Understand your surgery: Ask the doctor and surgeon how long the surgery will take, what will happen afterward, and how you can expect to feel during recovery.

Patients often notice errors: The staff will be grateful, especially if it helps avoid a serious mistake, so if you notice something, speak up!

YOU CAN CHECK OUT YOUR HOSPITAL

It's important to be aware of how and why mistakes happen and to stay alert. The public can obtain information from a hospital's accreditation performance report on www.jcaho.org, the web site of the Joint Commission on Accreditation of Healthcare Organizations.

Don't Panic — You are Safer In An American Hospital Than In Any Other Medical Facility On Earth.
- Most caregivers are well trained and conscientious.
- The medical profession's ability to save and extend life, and to improve the quality of life for the chronically ill is nothing short of miraculous. This applies not just to extraordinary procedures like heart transplants, but also to our ability to prevent, diagnose, treat, and often cure diseases that only a generation ago were routinely fatal. (Wachter and Shojania)

A Comprehensive System Will Help You Do Your Part. It Will Involve:
- Setting up the record keeping system.
- Gathering information, and documenting treatment and care.
- Being consistent in entering data.
- Keeping everything in a designated place.
- Routine updating.
- Sharing your information with your health care providers.

Health Information Multiplies with Age

As you become older there is a greater need for a clear tracking system for your medical care. Even the famous baby boomers have entered the phase of their lives where many are suddenly faced with a serious or chronic illness, adding to their already heavy load of putting their children through graduate school while being caretakers for their elderly parents.

Benefits of a Practical System

Having a clear system in place will help you deal with the increased complications. It will help you keep track of appointments, multiple physicians or changes in healthcare providers, medications, tests and procedures and their results, hospitalizations, out-patient treatment, insurance, and overall health costs. Once the system is set up you will find you can use it to access accurate information quickly.

With all pertinent information in one place, you, or someone who helps you, can document and coordinate all aspects of your health care. The peace of mind from knowing everything needed is at hand is an added bonus. It is especially important, in case of an emergency, that all your health information be accessed as soon as possible.

Patient as Consumer

Traditionally patients trusted their doctor to get them through each medical episode. The doctor made all the decisions and gave instructions not information. Today, when our doctor has evolved into a "primary care physician" who is assisted by numerous "healthcare professionals," we become so bombarded with information that our only choice is to participate in the process.

One obvious example of this is that drug companies are more and more marketing directly to the patient. Their assumption is that the patient as consumer is becoming more aware and more discerning. It is also one more indicator that patients need to take more and more responsibility for record keeping so they can be "educated" consumers.

Regarding medical treatment the watchword is "buyer beware." The more experience you have with the medical profession—one doctor after another, multiple doctors treating a serious or chronic condition, tests, procedures, hospitalization/s—the more you realize that as a patient you cannot remain passive. You are responsible for being informed and the best way to do that is to keep track of your own medical history.

First Step — Resolve to Take Control

Start by making the important decision to take responsibility for your own health. After that it will be you, the patient, who is taking the most active role in your own health care.

Partnership

The next step will be to establish a working partnership with your doctor and other health care practitioners. To do this you must first vow to become well informed and then ask your doctor to work *with* you, not just for you. Your doctor will greatly appreciate having a patient who can be relied upon to participate fully in decision making and treatment. Use this book to create your own personal knowledge base so you can use it as the foundation for the partnership.

Gathering and Analyzing Relevant Medical Information

As you begin to take more and more responsibility for your own health, you will realize the most crucial aspect is actually the most challenging, and that is to keep a clear and simple record of how you're doing. Recording basic information and using simple systems will keep you well informed and knowledgeable about your own personal health.

Once Upon a Time

In the old days, if we felt sick, we went to our family doctor, told him our symptoms, did what he told us, and got well. If we were really sick he would even come to our house. Only those of us over a certain age know this was once a reality and not just a fairy tale. Now we carefully scrutinize the health care providers we once trusted implicitly: After all, one of the 98,000 people who die from medical mistakes each year could be you or me!

Today

Now we rely on a series of primary physicians. Our current doctor is most likely to be in a group practice, which means we may or may not get our own primary in an emergency or weekend situation. When we move or change jobs or change insurance, we usually have to change doctors. And when our doctors retire or when they move their office, or reorganize their practice, we patients must adjust.

Paper Explosion

Because of the advances in medical technology, the increase in the number of specialists, and the patient's growing awareness and higher expectations, the amount of paperwork has mushroomed. With this information overload, doctors are not always receiving, in a timely manner, the reports or results they need from emergency rooms, labs, hospitals, other doctors, and diagnostic centers.

Getting Lost in Two Languages—Hard Copies and Computers

It's a fact of life today that things often get overlooked or even lost, with resulting delays, confusion, and even grievous errors. A major cause of this problem is that in addition to being kept in manila files, our records are now being kept simultaneously or separately on computer. Elaborate systems are set up to make sure there is communication between the two, but as of now there just aren't enough "translators" to go around. All the more reason for us to assume responsibility ourselves.

Preservation of Information Equals Self-Preservation

Who has the most to lose if information slips through the cracks? You do! Careful keeping of your own records is a way to make sure all medical information is stored safely, and is strong insurance against mistakes. If you acquire copies of all office visit notes, lab test results, hospital summaries, X-rays, etc., it guarantees key information does not go missing.

Your Doctor Also Wants to Know Everything You Know

It is extremely important to make available that part of your medical history that *only you can provide*. This includes any major medical conditions, family history, known allergies, medications and supplements. It would also include any tracking the doctor may ask you to do such as recording daily blood pressure, weight, blood sugar, etc. Insurance and financial information needs to be kept up to date as well. Your doctor will grow to rely on you for the information only you can provide. *Keeping Healthy by Keeping Track* is offered as a way for you to gather information to add to what your doctor already knows about you.

Acquiring and Storing Medical Information

We will walk you through gathering your medical information in a simple and systematic way. We will give examples of emergency information to keep by the phone, in the car, in your purse and wallet, at your neighbor's house, and at work. We will show how to keep your own charts and journals. We will offer a manageable storage and retrieval system. We will also give you hints to help you keep it all straight without its becoming one more enormous chore.

The more information you collect and process, the more self-knowledge you will have. You will better understand the procedures recommended by your medical practitioners, and you will be in a position to help make the important decisions and to monitor their implementation.

Establishing the Doctor — Patient Partnership

Your partnership will be strong if you truly commit yourself to becoming an expert on the state of your own health and if you make it clear you are taking responsibility for doing all you can to keep yourself as healthy as possible. The more carefully and accurately you record and transmit information, the more likely your doctor will accept its validity, and use it when analyzing your medical conditions and prescribing treatment.

EXACTLY WHAT IT IS WE PLAN TO KEEP TRACK OF

General
- Medical Appointments Calendar
- Medical Addresses—health practitioners, medical personnel and medical sites

Doctor Visits
- Intake forms
- Office visit notes as well as instructions from the doctor
- Your own notes after a doctor's visit
- Referrals

Specialists
- Consultation reports from other doctors and/or specialists

Patient Supplied Info
- Emergency information
- Medications list
- Personal health history
- Immunizations
- History of allergies
- Family health history
- Ongoing logs, journals, information sheets

Medications
- Prescriptions, over-the-counter drugs, vitamins, herbs, supplements

Labs and Testing
- Lab reports
- X-ray reports
- Actual test results
- Typed summaries

Hospitals
- Hospital discharge summaries

Insurance
- Private insurance
- Social Security

Finances
- Invoices, receipts, general financial papers

Legal Matters
- Advance directive (living will), power of attorney, will, etc.

Serious Health Conditions—Samples of Tracking
- Diabetes
- Cancer
- Allergies
- Heart Disease

THE RED NOTEBOOK–WHAT YOU WILL NEED TO GET STARTED

Address Book

Although we offer address pages to use in your Red Notebook, most people find it more convenient to keep their medical numbers in their usual Address Book. We suggest putting a red dot in front of medical people and places for quicker access.

Calendar

We also offer a calendar page for use in your Red Notebook, but we think your usual pocket or purse calendar is probably more efficient, especially if you red-dot the medical appointments to draw attention to them. The calendar is also an efficient way to track your pain level or how you're feeling by drawing faces each day.

Red Notebook

In your red notebook you will keep copies of all reports, notes, medications, side effects, informational pamphlets, etc. When any section of your red notebook becomes too full, you can transfer the oldest half of the information to your permanent health files. A dated zip-log bag makes a good file and allows for easy retrieval.

YOUR RED NOTEBOOK = YOUR PERSONAL HEALTH RECORD

Using a 3-ring binder as your **Red Notebook** you can design your own personal health organizer. It will be the central place you keep current health records, pending treatments and follow-up.

Your **Red Notebook** will become your personal health record.
With it you will be able to:
- Describe your current health status.
- Record symptoms, pain and side effects.
- Track your treatment and results.
- Schedule doctor appointments and scheduled tests.
- List office visit questions and record answers.
- Request copies of your doctor visits, lab reports, and test results,
- Store important material to read later.
- Document all key events of hospitalizations.
- Keep up with insurance paperwork.
- Access legal documents — advance directive, power of attorney, and will.
- Become more knowledgeable and self-confident.
- Form a successful partnership with your doctors.
- Make meaningful decisions about your own health care.

SETTING UP YOUR OWN RED NOTEBOOK

The backbone of your record keeping system, will be a red, flexible 3-ring binder. It will hold your entire tracking system. We suggest red because it will be easy to find and grab in case of an emergency. It will keep all basic information together in one compact container. Think of it as your own private medical reference book. It will always be there when you need it. And you will soon find yourself getting in the habit of taking it to every medical appointment.

Name your notebook only if you feel so compelled. Lillian did. She named it Ruby after Dorothy's slippers in The Wizard of Oz. She found out very quickly that people liked the name and remembered it. "It feels a little silly to remind the doctor's receptionist that Ruby needs a copy of my latest lab work, but she always complies with a smile."

WHAT YOU WILL NEED

- A red, 3-ring binder

- Copies of the charts you think you'll need to get started

- A color-coded table of contents — a set of notebook dividers made by Avery and available at Staples. It comes in either alphabetical order or with numbers. Remember, color helps to find information fast.

- 6 clear dividers with pockets to hold:
  - Pending items
  - Insurance materials
  - Financial items
  - Legal items – Advance Directive, Power of Attorney, Will
  - Completed items to be filed – Keep every scrap of paper that has any relevance at all to your medical care and remember to keep the latest information in front.
  - A complete set of blank charts to use for copies.

- Zip-lock bags for long term storage

As soon as your notebook is set up put the following in the appropriate sections:
- Pending medical business — anything current
- Primary Physician information — addresses, phone numbers, scheduled appointments, etc.
- Insurance info — private insurance and/or Social Security
- Financial info — current invoices and receipts
- A completely separate section of charts and information for any chronic or serious condition

The System is Simple and Self-evident.
Once you gather all your medical information and begin to put it in order, it will become obvious as to how it works. Ultimately you will individualize the system to meet your own personal needs. The point is to keep it simple so it's easy, and to be consistent so it becomes automatic.

TECHNOLOGY IS A BIG HELP FOR KEEPING TRACK

1. **Internet** access through your own computer would be very useful and convenient. Otherwise you can go online at your local library. Because so many people do have Internet access we have included a wide selection of Web Sites in the Resources section at the back of the book. You will find invaluable information on the Internet including:
   - Definitions of medical terms & abbreviations
   - Latest research
   - How to understand test results
   - Specialty centers
   - Information in Spanish
   - World health issues for travelers

2. **Copier** access will allow you to make any needed copies of charts. Libraries and stationery supply stores offer copiers for public use.

3. **Laminator** access will help preserve your emergency information sheets.

It's your system. Set it up to suit the way you think. We've included way more information and provided many more charts than any one individual will need or use. Select what's most useful and set the rest aside for possible later use. Remember, if you come up with a "better way" be sure to share it with us so we can include it in a future edition of *Keeping Healthy by Keeping Track*.

Note: Tape small items to 8 1/2" X 11" paper so they're easier to file.

GATHER PAST MEDICAL RECORDS ONLY IF YOU FEEL IT'S ESSENTIAL

As you begin to establish a new relationship with your doctor, you will quickly compile a complete medical record. You will gather more information and pay closer attention with each office visit, lab test, or other medical interaction. In no time you will find that you have a clear picture of you medical history and your current medical condition.

However, if you think it's necessary for you to refer to past records as well, you can request a copy of your complete medical file from your primary doctor. State laws require them to provide it. It might take weeks to receive it and you will probably have to pay a fee. When you make your request ask about charges and how soon you will receive your copy. Be sure to request that the copies be clear and readable.

Note: For your information, the authors did not feel the need to seek out past records. Once we started keeping better track we realized we had sufficient information to feel completely informed.

YOUR RED NOTEBOOK / SUGGESTED CONTENTS   Section

PART 1
DOCTOR PATIENT PARTNERSHIP

Note: Be sure you have copies of all blank charts before using.

Building a Partnership

Building a first rate working relationship is crucial to an effective doctor-patient partnership. Creating that relationship requires mutual respect and a free flow of information both ways. Doctors and patients must keep each other informed, when things are going well and when there are concerns. It's important for both the doctor and the patient to lend willing support to one another and to avoid threatening each other's territory. Each must respect the role played by the other so both parties can focus on their common goal—the patient's health.

A New Way of Viewing the Doctor–Patient Connection

The doctor-patient relationship is a serious one, usually subtle as well as complicated. Today we patients know more—about our bodies, about health in general, and about the medical profession. We are no longer willing to just do as we are told. We must have a say in what happens to us.

Are You Ready to Do Your Part?

Ask yourself what you must do to create this new relationship? What information must you bring to the table? Are you willing to make the effort? What will the doctor want? What will help the doctor help you? Are you ready to meet the doctor's needs?

Start by Making A List

Picture the kind of relationship you wish to have with your primary doctor and all your other health-care providers. It will take time for you to clarify what it is you want. Making a list is a useful strategy. Jot down your thoughts as you go. The clearer you are, the better you will be able to communicate your ideas. Be sure to include everything that is important to you. Add whatever new ideas occur to you later. If you want to be sure your doctor is clear about your expectations you might want to give her a copy of the list you create.

You Might Come Up With A List Similar to This:

- I want to participate in all decisions relating to my own health.
- I want clear and accurate information.
- I want to be treated with courtesy and respect at all times.
- I want to have a person I trust participate in all phases of my care, should I need that assistance.
- I want reasonable access to my primary physician and any specialists.
- I want to know the role of everyone involved in my health care and their credentials.
- I want a clear evaluation of any serious condition before any tests or procedures are started.
- I always want to feel free to ask why.
- I want to know how a test will help, as well as the costs and the risks.
- I want to know what my choices are, including the choice to do nothing.
- I want the option of freely seeking a second opinion.
- I want to be able to refuse any drug, test, procedure, or treatment if I so choose.
- I want itemized bills so that I can check them over myself, even if my insurance is paying most of the costs.
- I want access to all my medical records should I choose to see them, and to ask for copies should I want them.
- I want prompt transfer of my records should I move or change doctors.

1a   MAKE A LIST OF WHAT YOU WANT IN A PARTNERSHIP

Things I Want in a Partnership

_____

_____

_____

_____

_____

_____

_____

_____

_____

_____

_____

_____

_____

_____

_____

_____

_____

_____

_____

_____

_____

_____

_____

_____

_____

_____

_____

_____

_____

_____

_____

_____

WHAT WILL YOU BRING TO THE PARTNERSHIP?

Whether you realize it or not, there are things that only you can tell your doctor. Pledge to make every effort to know and understand your own body. Although the doctor must always take the lead in a medical situation, you have a unique vantage point from which to offer valid information. You possess a wide range of knowledge that only you can offer.

The More Information the Better

Start to use the library, the Internet, the media and information booklets from the doctor's office to add to your health knowledge. The charts and suggestions in this book will help you to collect and organize specific and detailed information. The more carefully and accurately you record and transmit information about yourself, the more likely the doctor will accept its validity and add it to what she has already learned. She can then use this fuller picture to analyze your condition and prescribe treatment.

You Can Play a Stronger Role

As you gather information you will also gain increased awareness. Your increased knowledge will enable you to better understand the recommendations of your doctor and help you monitor procedures and recommendations. You will notice that as you become better informed your doctor will be more willing to share more detailed information with you. She will communicate her diagnosis clearly and describe the treatment options available, then you can make the best choice together.

From The Doctor's Point of View

Once you're clear about the partnership you seek and what you yourself must bring to the table, it's time to think about it from the doctor's point of view. It's important to respect the doctor as a highly trained and experienced medical professional. In analyzing your condition and recommending treatment your doctor can and must take the lead.

What the Doctor Will and Won't Do

The doctor will answer your concerns, but if you want the detailed knowledge only gained in medical school you'll have to enroll yourself. The doctor will be glad to see you taking notes but won't wait forever while you write down every word. The doctor will give you a clear explanation, but not an all-day seminar on diabetes. If you fumble with your newly acquired medical vocabulary and concepts, the doctor will be patient, but only up to a point. Be reasonable in what you expect.

Communication is Key

Learning some good basic communication skills will help. Ask your questions in plain English and the doctor will respond in plain English. Be careful. If you begin to salt your conversation with medical terminology you will either embarrass yourself as you show your incorrect or limited knowledge, or you might succeed in convincing your doctor you know more than you do, and miss out on more careful explanations.

Practice What You Might Say

Is the doctor rushed, inattentive, going through the motions, going too fast? Rather than getting huffy or clamming up, be friendly—but candid.

- Could you slow down a bit?
- Would you write that down for me?
- Would you repeat that for me?
- How do you spell that.
- I think I need a bit more time to be clear on what you're telling me.
- May I tell you what I understand about what you've just told me?
- I seem to need more time for this to sink in. Should I come back?

SETTING UP THE PARTNERSHIP

Make a Special Appointment to Talk with Your Doctor

You must be prepared to take the lead in establishing a new relationship with your doctor. You might want to sit down and explain what it is you want. If so, schedule an appointment for that specific purpose. During this visit your goal will be to let your doctor know you intend to become more fully informed and willing to assume full responsibility for shared decision making. Bring your notebook and describe briefly how you plan to keep track. Make sure your doctor knows how much you respect her and how much you appreciate the care you are currently receiving. Let her know you plan to take more responsibility for your health, and that you think keeping track will help you do that. If you would like a copy of your past records, now is the time to make the request. (Make sure your doctor doesn't think you're doing this so you can change doctors, or to get a secret second opinion.)

Or Just Start Behaving Differently

An alternative plan is simply to begin acting in a different manner. If you're clear about what you want, you will be able to communicate it clearly without alienating or irritating the doctor or her staff. It will be pretty obvious you're taking a more active role and a more informed interest, and that your doctor/patient relationship has reached a different level if you:

- Always bring a written list of concerns.
- Take notes.
- Ask clear questions.
- Request copies of office visit notes.
- Request copies of lab reports.
- Bring your Red Notebook, carefully organized, and refer to it in response to requests for information.

In Any Case, From Now On Always Ask for Copies of:

- Your doctor's notes after every visit.
- Reports from specialists.
- Lab reports.
- Results of all other evaluations authorized by your doctor.

Note: Do Unto Others… Be Nice
Most interactions with your primary physician will take place in the office and with the office staff. It's always appropriate to be pleasant, respectful and cooperative. Be patient, smile, learn people's names, say please and thank you.

Becoming Familiar with Office Routine

The people you meet in the office are important. Become acquainted with how the office works and who the key people are. The receptionist will ask you for some general information—your insurance carrier, your health history, etc. The doctor's nurse may weigh you and take vital signs and ask some preliminary questions. The doctor will usually speak with her before seeing you. You will check with the receptionist once more when you leave—to handle payment details and make your next appointment. Take note of each person's name and job.

10-15 Minute Appointments Are the Norm

It doesn't sound like much time but it is adequate for most office visits and includes time to state your concerns, be examined and diagnosed, to write prescriptions or to make arrangements for further tests or treatments, and to answer any further questions. If you think you might need more time, say so when you call to schedule. It might surprise you to know doctors typically allow about 30 seconds for their patients to talk before interrupting them. If you don't want to feel rushed, be prepared.

Bring All Your Prescription Medications to Every Visit

Medical personnel prefer to see the original containers rather than read a list you prepare. A zip-lock bag with your name on it is useful for bringing your medicines, in their original bottles, to every office appointment. Also bring a list of any over-the-counter drugs, vitamins, or herbs you might be taking regularly or occasionally. If you are on a diet, seeing other doctors, or receiving alternative therapy, be sure to let your doctor know; don't wait to be asked.

Cancellations

If you can't keep an appointment, call to cancel as soon as possible. Give at least 24 hours if you can. Courtesy goes both ways. Some offices charge if they don't receive a 24 hour notice of a cancellation.

Emergencies

If you don't already know, ask the receptionist how they expect you to interact with their office in case of emergency. *Keep the information with your insurance cards—either in your purse or wallet.*

Seeing the Doctor

A visit to a doctor is an important and sometimes crucial event. We generally take it quite seriously and so do doctors and their staffs. Remember that any good patient-doctor partnership consists of shared effort towards good patient health, and is based on good communication.

Before You Go — Write It Down

You can best include everything pertinent if you make notes beforehand. List your symptoms, their severity and when they occur. Make note of your pain level if any. Include everything you can think of, even if it feels unimportant. Ask close family or friends if they noticed anything significant. The more information you provide the doctor, the better her analysis of the problem. Organize all the information you gather into a concise statement of your concern so that you can present it clearly and efficiently.

Clear Communication Is Essential
Listen carefully to your doctor and get clarification as needed. Jot down the diagnosis, treatment and follow-up plan. Ask the doctor to repeat, speak up, or slow down—whatever you need to make sure you understand. The doctor is not a mind reader. If you don't understand, ask for clarification. If you have vague or serious doubts, or if you don't agree, say so. If you feel uncertain about your diagnosis or treatment plan, speak up. If you have a worry—Is this serious? Will my children be at risk? Is it cancer? Will it leave a scar?—ask. You'll probably be reassured, and you've let the doctor know how to help you.

Many people have difficulty thinking on the spot, so your doctor won't be surprised if you remember something important later and call back for clarification. A clear understanding of all the issues relating to your own health will better prepare you to participate effectively in important decision making.

> *Note: Not knowing does not mean you are stupid. On the contrary, asking questions tells the doctor you are a very smart patient, willing to understand your illness and participate in treatment.*

Do What the Doctor Says
It is a curious fact that most people do not follow their doctor's instructions. Unless you have already communicated your reluctance to do so or your intention not to, it makes sense to follow the doctor's instructions. It wastes time and money, both yours and the doctor's, if you do not do what is recommended. With your new-found skill as a true partner, you will find it easier now to follow your doctor's advice. When you help make the decisions, you have a vested interest in a positive outcome.

Do Your Part
- Get required immunizations.
- Get appropriate health screenings.
- Don't smoke.
- Stay fit; exercise.
- Eat right.
- Get a good night's sleep.
- Use alcohol in moderation.
- Do not use illegal drugs, period.
- Take care of your teeth.
- Smile.
- Be positive.
- Be happy.

Remember Names and Faces—If you want to be treated like an important individual then treat the doctor and her staff like important individuals. Learn their names; understand their different responsibilities. Greet them by name. Introduce or re-introduce yourself at every encounter. Almost everyone in a medical setting wears a nametag or an I.D. on a cord, so it's simple to read a name, make eye contact, and say something friendly using their name.

Professional vs Personal—Doctors' offices are becoming more informal, with staff usually referring to themselves and their co-workers by their first names, the doctor being the exception. In general, take your cue from the staff. If the receptionist introduces herself as Nancy with no last name given, then obviously you are free to call her Nancy.

Calling the Doctor

We usually call to set up or verify an appointment. We also call when we don't know what to do, or when we're not sure if we should come to the office or go to the emergency room. We call when the office is closed and we're uncertain as to how serious the problem is. In short, we call when we have an urgent medical concern. Still—it's best to make some notes before we call, even if it's for an emergency. Have your calendar and notepad ready. Be concise, because you're more than likely going to get a receptionist or answering service.

- Tell what's wrong and describe the symptoms in no more than two sentences.
- Tell what you've already done and what you think caused the problem.
- Ask no more than 2 or 3 questions.
- Ask the receptionist when you can expect your call to be returned.
- Tell what you plan to do while you're waiting.
- Have a pharmacy phone number ready if one may be needed.
- Recognize that most conditions may require an office visit for the most accurate diagnosis and treatment.

Note: You would be amazed how many people call, ask the doctor to return their call, then say, "I'll be out all day." If it's urgent, make sure you can be reached.

Most people find their primary care physician by default (only choice in town), through a friend (you'll love him), through HMO lists (there were only two listed and the one I wanted was on maternity leave), etc. If you should be one of the fortunate few who actually have a choice of doctors, get ready to make your best choice.

Word of mouth is still the most common and most reliable way to find a good doctor for you and your family. Ask family, friends, neighbors, and fellow workers for suggestions. Most likely they will also know if their nominee is accepting new patients.

The words family doctor conjure up wonderfully warm images of midnight rides through snowdrifts in a horse drawn sleigh driven by a wise and friendly doctor who rushes in to save us at the very last minute. Today's doctor is called a Primary Physician or Health Care Provider and never (or almost never) makes house calls. However, the basic image is still the same— someone we can count on when an illness strikes and we're completely terrified. We still think of our doctor as an individual. If he is part of a team, then he's the captain in our mind.

The most common replacement for the all-around General Practitioner is either a Family Practitioner or an Internist. Once we make our choice of Primary Caregiver we generally rely on them to recommend any needed specialists.

- A Family Practitioner (FP) has a specialty in Family Medicine. He has earned an M.D. or D.O. degree, completed a year's internship, and done a 3-year residency (that covers internal medicine, gynecology, obstetrics, pediatrics, minor surgery, preventive medicine, etc.). They then take a board exam in family practice.
- An Internist has also completed a 3-year residency and in addition has passed a rigorous examination to become board certified. His training is focused on all the organ systems of adults such as gastrointestinal tract, liver, kidney, heart, etc.
- Two other significant primary caregivers—Nurse Practitioner (N.P.) and Physician's Assistant (P.A.)—work closely with a physician. They have a great deal of autonomy, but check in with the doctor if there is an unusual finding or if they have a question.

Verifying Credentials
You might want to use the book *Official ABMS Directory of Board-Certified Medical Specialists* to verify that the doctor you are considering is board-certified. You'll also want to know where he received his medical training and where he did his residency training, as well as how long he has been practicing. Believe it or not, an MD can legally present himself as a specialist without having any training in that specialty, so you might do well to check it out, especially if the doctor you're considering is unknown to you.

After You Have a Few Candidates
Call the office and find out if the #1 doctor you are considering is accepting new patients. Be sure to let the receptionist know who recommended you. Although most doctors don't do this (they are not paid for it) ask to schedule an interview visit. You'll be taking notes during the visit but since people usually size new people up in under ten seconds, be especially careful to notice how you are responding.

Finding a Doctor or Re-Evaluating Your Current One

Because her role in your life will be so important you must choose your Primary Caregiver wisely. You are seeking a doctor you can entrust with a most precious possession, your health. Office staff can answer some of your questions, but there are many, many things to find out and you'll want to hear some of the more important answers directly from your potential doctor.

SOME THINGS YOU WILL NEED TO FIND OUT

Highly recommended? Who praised this doctor and for what qualities? Are there any red flags? Keep a plus and minus list.

Credentials: Do enough research to make sure you know her qualifications.

Experience: Where has she practiced, for how long, and with what kind of patients? Remember young doctors have the most up-to-date training, although older ones are more experienced.

Availability: Will she return your calls, see you promptly when you have an appointment?

Emergency or serious concerns: Will your call be answered promptly? Will she respond quickly if called on your behalf from an Emergency Room?

Emergency service: Does the doctor respond to the emergency center nearest you?

Routine Visits: How much time is allowed? How far ahead must you call for a routine appointment?

May you bring a relative or friend? You might need a second pair of ears at some point.

Is she in a group practice? Who are the other doctors and what are their qualifications? How likely are you to be treated by a partner?

Office personnel: Does the doctor work with Nurse Practitioners or Physician Assistants? These health professionals have special training in managing minor and routine health problems. They can often see you sooner, spend more time with you, and help you just as well as a doctor can.

Fees schedule, cancellation charges: You need to know all costs.

Insurance cooperation: Will the office staff fill out forms and provide needed information?

Prescriptions: What are the procedures for securing the best drugs at the lowest cost?

Hospital affiliation: Is it reasonably convenient?

Talk about yourself: The doctor wants to get to know you, too.

Diagnoses: Will you be filled in on the total picture?

Treatment decisions: Will you make them together after she lets you know the benefits and risks (and costs) of each option?

Records and test results: How will you obtain copies?

Willingness to partner with you: Be clear about the relationship you want with your Primary Health Care Provider. Will she work with you?

Some Things You Will Need To Find Out
- Accepting new patients: _____
- Recommended by: _____
- Credentials: _____
- Experience: _____
- Availability: _____
- Procedure for routine visits: _____
- May I bring a relative or friend? _____
- Group practice: _____
- Key office personnel: _____
- Procedures for phone consults: _____
- Liaison with nearby emergency service: _____
- Fee schedule, charges: _____
- Insurance cooperation & forms: _____
- Low-cost prescriptions: _____
- Hospital affiliation: _____
- Tell about yourself: _____
- Diagnosis—full disclosure: _____
- Joint treatment decisions: _____
- Copies of records & test results: _____
- Willingness to partner with you: _____

After The Interview, Evaluate Your Candidate.
- Was the doctor relaxed and welcoming, or did you feel rushed?

_____

_____

- Could you understand what she said, or was she talking over your head?

_____

_____

- Did she listen carefully to your questions, and answer straightforwardly?

_____

_____

- Did you feel you could become good partners?

_____

_____

Other Notes

_____

_____

_____

_____

_____

_____

_____

_____

Go Prepared

The doctor's first question is usually, "How are you doing?" He's not just saying, "Hi, how are you?" he's asking for information. Keep a simple ongoing record of any symptoms—headaches, pain, discomfort, etc.

Pain Scale

Doctors and nurses use either a "0-5 scale," a "1-10 scale" or "faces" when rating a patient's pain. Ask what scale your doctor uses and then describe your pain accordingly.

Do Research

Do some research ahead of time and make an informed guess as to what your problem might be. Doctors recognize that patients have excellent insight into what is happening with their own bodies.

Put It in Writing

Fill in *Chart 1c, Office Visit Form,* with as much information as you can, include the questions you want answered. List your most important concerns. Be clear and concise.

Ask for Clarification

If you don't understand or you're just not sure, be sure to say so. Don't hesitate to say no to anything you're not clear about—medications, tests, procedures, referrals, etc.

Take a Relative or Friend

If you need backup to understand the doctor's instructions, make sure you have someone you trust go with you. Ask her to take notes and help you remember all the important items.

Doctor's Notes

Ask for a copy of your doctor's notes which are usually being made during your visit. Look at them quickly and ask for clarification if you can't read them. Note: Not everyone will have these. Many people dictate them. Increasingly these will be done on computer using voice recognition, in which case you can request they be copied to your email address.

Prescriptions

Make sure all instructions and prescriptions are in writing before you leave the office.

Make Your Own Notes

After the visit, write down in detail everything that is important. You can then refer to your notes, and to the doctor's, to make sure you remember everything.

Follow Up

If you have any question about what you are supposed to do, call the office. Patients commonly call back to double check.

Update You Records At Home

Record all new information on your charts, making special note of any changes.

1c   OFFICE VISIT   **Appointment Date** _____
                                           Next Appointment _____

Be prepared. Fill in this form before going to the doctor so you won't forget important items.

Doctor _____   Phone _____
Address _____
_____

Reason/s for Visit
(routine, yearly physical, accident, emergency, illness, etc.) _____
_____
Present complaint & onset _____
_____
Symptoms & how often _____
_____
Describe pain (shooting, sharp, localized, aching, throbbing, burning, deep, surface, sharp, dull)
_____
Concerns & questions _____
_____
_____

Office Test Results
Height _____   Blood Pressure _____   Temp _____
Weight _____   Blood Sugar _____   Other _____

Doctor's Analysis and Instructions
Diagnosis
_____
Prognosis
_____
Prescription/s
_____
Tests
_____
Recommendations
_____
Follow Up
_____

*Note: After your office visit, staple any information you receive to this chart.
Process all relevant information into your Red Notebook charts. Record all items
such as weight, blood pressure, blood sugar, etc., as well as more significant
information and instructions.*

Test/Procedure

Name of test/procedure. _____

Why is it recommended? _____

What are the alternatives? _____

Where can you obtain additional information? _____

_____

Side Effects

Pain or discomfort during test? _____

Afterwards? _____

Risk? _____

Results

What are the results? _____

How common are incorrect results? (false positive or false negative) _____

Should we automatically re-test to make sure? _____

Treatment

Description of treatment. _____

Effects and duration of treatment. _____

What happens without the treatment? _____

Costs

How much does the test cost? _____

What will insurance cover? _____

Is the test too costly or too risky? _____

Be forthright

State your concerns; share your fears. _____

_____

Satisfy yourself that your doctor has a total picture of your health. _____

Be sure you're clear about all medications and treatments. _____

Give a Clear Yes or No _____

If Yes—Cooperate

Follow all instructions to the letter. _____

Make daily notes. _____

Keep your doctors and other caregivers informed. _____

If there are unusual or painful effects, holler! _____

Notes:

OFFICE VISIT / SPECIALIST

Your Primary Physician is probably not a GP (General Practitioner) but a specialist—possibly an Internist. This means she has had extended training including a 3-year residency in Internal Medicine, has passed a rigorous examination and has become Board Certified.

There are more and more specialists, and sub-specialists, these days, doctors who are trained in an even more specific area such as arthritis, cardiology, oncology, obstetrics, etc. It usually costs more to see a specialist, and the tests and treatment they prescribe are usually more expensive as well.

It's unlikely you yourself will initiate contact with a specialist. The main reason is that, for most of us, our medical lives are dependent on HMO's which means your insurance probably doesn't cover your seeing a specialist without a recommendation from your Primary Physician.

Also, very few of us have the knowledge or skill to seek out and select the best person to handle a specific problem. Things are further complicated by the extraordinary waiting time to see a specialist, sometimes as long as three months. And many specialty practices are closed to all but referrals from specific doctors.

Given all of the above reasons for not having direct access, it's still important to gather as much information about specialists as possible. Knowing the best doctors, the ones your friends and acquaintances admire and rely on, is just one more way of being an informed medical consumer. Keep a list of the ones your doctor refers you to, and any others you hear positive things about. Keep them in your back pocket "just in case."

There is specific information you will want to have at hand, when you do begin to see a specialist. The same kinds of things you have learned about your Primary Physician—probably over time—will be important for you to know—all at once. Having basic information ahead of time will allow you to spend more of your actual appointment time addressing your serious health problem.

You can learn quite a bit about the specialist from your Primary Physician's office, so be sure and ask. In addition, call the specialist's office and find out when is a good time to get specific information on the phone. They might offer to email or fax you information. They might ask you to come early to see a film in their office. You might look up their specialty on the Internet and see what you can learn there. The better informed you are, the more you will be able to understand your diagnosis and take part in the treatment plan.

Your Primary Physician will keep in touch with the results and recommendations from the specialist. If you have any questions or concerns be sure to ask your Primary Physician. She will be in close touch with the specialist and will be able to discuss the results and recommendations with you. If you are hospitalized you might be visited and/or treated by both doctors, but this is happening less and less. Many primary care doctors are now referring their patients to Hospitalists—usually internists, pediatricians or FPs—who only see patients in the hospital.

Use your usual Office Visit Form (Chart 1c) to prepare for your visit to the specialist.
Make sure you have all of the following additional information:

Referring physician_____
Reason for referral _____

_____
Specialist_____
Specialty _____
Address _____
Phone_____
Hospital/s (where s/he practices) _____
Board Certification _____
Hospital of Residency_____
Office contact person _____
How busy is the practice?_____
How long will it be before your first appointment; how soon will you be re-seen_____

_____
Does the office run on time?_____
Insurance process—referral required, method of payment, etc. _____

_____
Information the specialist might need ahead of time:
   • From you _____

   • From your doctor_____

Lab reports needed ahead of visit_____

Who gets copies of reports from specialist?
   • You_____
   • Your primary physician _____
   • Other specialists _____
   • Others in practice _____
Additional information _____

_____

*Note: Keep a list of specialists who are great even if you don't currently need them.
Maybe you will. Listen when your friends praise their hip guy, their knee guy, their
aunt's cataract man, etc.*

PART 2
BASIC CHARTS FOR KEEPING TRACK

This section contains 14 charts covering background information and ongoing monitoring of key aspects of your health. These charts are the foundation of your record keeping system.

Note: Be sure to make copies of all blank charts before using.

2a   EMERGENCY AND MEDICAL NUMBERS

- Make copies before using
- Keep laminated copy in family cars
- Keep laminated copy by home and work phones
- Give laminated copies to neighbors
- Give laminated copies to babysitters

Family Name _____   **Home Phone** _____

Address_____

Family Members   **Birth Dates**   **Work/School Phone**

Name _____   _____   _____
Name _____   _____   _____
Name _____   _____   _____
Name _____   _____   _____

Emergency Contacts	**Name**	**Address**	**Phone**
Neighbor/Friend	_____	_____	_____
Neighbor/Friend	_____	_____	_____
Emergency	_____	_____	_____
Poison Control Center	_____	_____	_____
Fire Department	_____	_____	_____
Nearest Hospital	_____	_____	_____
Preferred Hospital	_____	_____	_____
Taxi	_____	_____	_____
Emergency Shelter	_____	_____	_____
Nearest Pharmacy	_____	_____	_____
All-night Pharmacy	_____	_____	_____

Doctor_____   **Phone**_____

Address_____

_____
_____
_____
_____
_____
_____

Other Medical Resources

_____
_____
_____
_____
_____

Update on your birthday.

HEALTH LOG

Use this Health Log to keep ongoing notes of all important medical events. Entries should answer the fact questions: *who, what, when, where, how and why*. Be sure to document:

Sudden Changes in the Following
- Sleep Patterns
- Appetite
- Digestion
- Sense of Time and Place
- Body Cycles
- Pain
- Mood
- Carrying Out Routine Tasks
- Memory
- Balance
- Energy
- Communication

Major or Chronic Illnesses: Cancer, diabetes, kidney disease, bladder or kidney infections, eyes, ears, nose, or skin problems, etc.

Surgeries: Scheduled or emergency. Always request a summary of your treatment records.

Hospitalizations: Routine or emergency.

Injuries: Especially broken bones and head injuries

Medications: A new prescription, change of medication, side effects of medications

Vitamins, Supplements, Over-the-counter Drugs

Contagious Diseases: Chicken pox, cholera, diphtheria, flu, hepatitis B, hepatitis C, HIV/Aids, malaria, measles, mumps, pneumonia, smallpox, tetanus, tuberculosis, typhoid, and yellow fever. Be sure to make note of all exposures in U.S. or foreign countries, particularly of actual diseases contracted.

Make Note of:
- High temperature
- All complaints and symptoms,
- Unusual reaction to food or exercise
- New diet or exercise program
- Irregular periods
- Severe cold or flu
- Specific or severe pain or discomfort
- Sudden weight loss or gain
- Specific advice from the doctor
- Change in usual health habits

Serious and Life Threatening Occurrences:
- Unconsciousness
- No pulse
- Bites
- Choking
- Heavy bleeding
- Hypothermia, over-heating
- Poisoning
- Allergic reactions
- Burns
- Shock or trauma

Away From Home: Be especially careful to document illnesses, accidents and injuries that occur while on vacations. Notes are particularly important when you are away from your usual health care personnel and facilities. Details are significant for follow-up by your primary care giver, especially for insurance purposes.

Name _____   Date of Birth _____

Date   **Event**

_____
_____
_____
_____
_____
_____
_____
_____
_____
_____
_____
_____
_____
_____
_____
_____
_____
_____
_____
_____
_____
_____
_____
_____
_____
_____
_____
_____
_____
_____
_____
_____
_____
_____
_____
_____
_____

Remember a log is sequential and ongoing. It answers the fact
questions—*who, what, when, where, how* and *why*.

• Use this calendar only for doctor visits, lab tests, screenings, procedures, scheduled surgery, etc.
• It will keep all medically related appointments in one place, on one sheet.
• It will give at one glance a snapshot of your yearly health activity.
• At the end of the year file it with your permanent record materials.

Medical Appointments   Name _____
                                                      Year _____

January	February	March	April
_____	_____	_____	_____
_____	_____	_____	_____
_____	_____	_____	_____
_____	_____	_____	_____
_____	_____	_____	_____
_____	_____	_____	_____
_____	_____	_____	_____
_____	_____	_____	_____
_____	_____	_____	_____

May	June	July	August
_____	_____	_____	_____
_____	_____	_____	_____
_____	_____	_____	_____
_____	_____	_____	_____
_____	_____	_____	_____
_____	_____	_____	_____
_____	_____	_____	_____
_____	_____	_____	_____
_____	_____	_____	_____

September	October	November	December
_____	_____	_____	_____
_____	_____	_____	_____
_____	_____	_____	_____
_____	_____	_____	_____
_____	_____	_____	_____
_____	_____	_____	_____
_____	_____	_____	_____
_____	_____	_____	_____

2d   MEDICAL ADDRESSES

Name	Address	Phone	Email

SIGNIFICANT HEALTH AND MEDICAL HISTORY

It is crucial to help your doctor create an accurate health picture of you as a patient. The more detailed information you provide, the better he can do his job of analyzing and recommending good health practices for you.

Significant Medical History

In order to provide essential background information, you will need to sit down and think back over your life in detail and pick out the significant health events. You also might need to ask relatives what they remember about your health, especially when you were young.

When documenting your Significant Medical History, try to think in chronological terms, starting with infancy, childhood, adolescence, young adulthood, middle age, retirement age, and more advanced years. Use approximate dates if you can't recall precisely.

Family History

Many health conditions are hereditary. Use the Family Health History in the next section to include significant health events for your parents, siblings and extended family.

Note: While it is very important to know your medical history, keep in mind the purpose for completing it is to provide accurate background information. Your main focus must be to create a clear and simple system so you can keep track now and in the future.

Name _____   Date of Birth_____

Current Health Profile
Include any health issues you currently have, and how they affect your life. List anything and everything that might be significant. Remember, you're trying to paint a total picture.

• Vital statistics   Blood type _____   Height _____   Weight _____   Blood pressure _____

　　　　　　　　　　Cholesterol _____   HDL _____   LDL _____   Triglycerides _____

• **Immediate Health Concerns** _____
_____
_____

• **Chronic/serious medical condition** _____
_____
_____

• **Allergies** _____
_____
_____

• **General health and hygiene habits** _____
_____
_____

• **Current stressors in your life** _____
_____
_____

• **Medications you are currently taking** _____
_____
_____

• **Herbal medicines, vitamins or supplements** _____
_____
_____

• **Continued use of over-the-counter medications** _____
_____
_____

• **Alternative medicine such as chiropractic or homeopathy** _____
_____
_____

Sit quietly and think about your past medical history; most relevant information will come back to you. Concentrate on the most outstanding health and medical events.

Make note of important contacts with healthcare providers so you won't have to rely on your memory. Most likely you'll be asked for this information again and again.

Name _____   Date of Birth _____

Include All Relevant Information:

- Emergency events
- Hospitalizations
- Major illnesses
- Surgeries

Date   **Event**

_____
_____
_____
_____
_____
_____
_____
_____
_____
_____
_____
_____
_____
_____
_____
_____
_____
_____
_____
_____
_____
_____
_____
_____
_____
_____
_____

Remember a log is sequential and ongoing. It answers the fact
questions—*who, what, when, where, how* and *why*.

Genetics

Because families share the same genetic makeup (DNA) family members have similar propensities for certain hereditary conditions. The big killers—cancer, heart disease, stroke, diabetes, and kidney disease—sometimes run in families. Some other diseases with a genetic component are Alzheimer's, glaucoma, osteoporosis, multiple sclerosis, allergies, schizophrenia, depression, sickle cell anemia, Tay-Sachs and hemophilia.

Lifestyle

Because they share the same physical space and similar lifestyle influences, family members are also prone to the same environmentally caused diseases, conditions or illnesses. Environment and lifestyle related conditions include tobacco and alcohol abuse, obesity radiation sickness, etc., and infectious diseases such as worms, tuberculosis, etc.

When filling out your Family Medical History it's important to include every serious health condition you can remember or research. The more information you can give your doctor, the more she can help you avoid serious problems arising out of family tendencies.

As you accumulate more and more information about your family's health, a clear pattern will emerge. Share the information with your doctor and together you will identify disease patterns and health risks.

Your doctor will discuss with you the many advances in medical treatment, and more important, help you develop *prevention techniques* so you can put a new spin on your heredity.

Choices

Three significant diseases—Type II diabetes, some cancers, and some aspects of heart disease—are more and more being thought of as *chosen diseases* rather than destiny diseases, because a healthier lifestyle (primarily a healthy diet, maintaining normal weight and regular exercise) is now known to prevent or forestall them.

Overall, the more information you have the more choices you have when it comes to managing hereditary health problems.

2g   FAMILY MEDICAL HISTORY

Name _____   Date of Birth _____

	Born	Died	Cause of Death	Diseases	Other
Sister/s					
Brother/s					
Mother					
Mother's Mother					
Mother's Father					
Mother's Sisters					
Mother's Brothers					
Father					
Father's Mother					
Father's Father					
Father's Sisters					
Father's Brothers					

Other Important Family Medical Information

_____

_____

_____

_____

_____

MEDICATIONS AND SUPPLEMENTS

These logs are provided to maintain a running list of medications and supplements used to combat physical and emotional discomfort or illness.

Medications log: We are terming medications all prescriptions or over-the-counter drugs taken by mouth or applied topically.

Supplements log: It's important to also make note of any herbs, vitamins or minerals you usually, or sometimes, take.

PHARMACY

Try to use only one drugstore to fill prescriptions. Make sure they have an automatic system in place that cross checks your medications to see they do not interfere with each other's efficacy.

Make a copy before handing over your prescription to the pharmacist.

Double check:
- With the druggist, compare the prescription bottle to your copy to make sure that the prescription you have received is what the doctor prescribed and that it is for the condition you have.
- Is your name correct on the prescription and on the bottle? If you have a somewhat common first or last name then use a middle initial also.
- Is the prescription name precisely the same?
- Is the dosage/frequency the same?
- Are the instructions clear?
- Is the information sheet enclosed? (Be aware of the generic and the brand names.)

Be alert to:
- Abbreviations
- Use of Latin
- Poor handwriting
- Similar names or similar sounding names
- Capital letters intermixed with numerals

Toxic pharmacology (also known as polypharmacy)—This is a term being used more and more to describe the increase in the number of prescriptions written for one individual (as high as 30) and the possible negative effect of drug interactions. It's something to be aware of and a reason for careful and periodic review if you are taking multiple medications.

Safety first—In order to prevent adverse drug reactions always refer to the medical information sheet when you start taking a new drug, herb, over-the-counter preparation, vitamin or supplement. Before you leave the drugstore, verify that there is information included that explains how the drug acts, describes any possible side effects, and warnings of negative interactions with other drugs or supplements.

Keep info sheets—Get in the habit of dating and keeping info sheets for future reference. Also keep the peel-off labels, handouts, or other package inserts from your pharmacy, all of which contain important information about your medications.

Store medications properly—Note the storage instructions given by the pharmacy or manufacturer.

Regularly review your medications. Make a list of all your medications and supplements and then bring the list along with everything in their original containers in a zip-lock bag to every doctor's visit. Include over-the-counter drugs, and herbs, vitamins and minerals. The physical presence of what you regularly use will be a gentle nudge for a careful review by the doctor or staff. It also lets them see if you've refilled a prescription, etc.

Take your medicine. If the doctor has prescribed it, it's important to follow her directions and take it as prescribed. Don't double the dose, set it aside before the full course is completed, or decide not to bother taking it without informing your doctor.

Never take someone else's prescribed medication without your doctor's permission.

Never take out-of-date medications without checking with your doctor first.

Keep an updated list of your meds in your wallet or purse in case of emergency. Include your current medications, vitamins and supplements, and any over-the-counter drugs you routinely take.

Questions to Ask Your Doctor About Prescriptions

   Name: What's it called? Check the spelling.

   Cost: Is it available in a generic form? Is it better to stick with the brand name?

   Dosage/Frequency: How much will I be taking? How often?

   When: Time of day? With or without food?

   Temperature Requirement: Refrigeration?

   Side Effects: What might occur? What to do if there's a problem?

   Drug Interactions: Is it OK with what I'm already taking?

   Restrictions: Alcohol? Foods?

   Problems: Whom do I call? How about after hours?

   Travel Tips: Keep all medicines in your carry-on bag. Bring extras.

MEDICATIONS SIDE EFFECTS

- Each patient may experience different side effects or none at all.
- Be aware of the known side effects for the medication/s you are taking and let your doctor know if you are experiencing any or all of them, and to what extent.
- Also know, you may be having side effects that aren't listed. You and your doctor together can try to discern the cause, and make your best guess as to whether it is the medication, a combination of medications or some other reason.
- Some patients study the written side effects given at the time of getting the prescription, and are unduly and erroneously influenced towards experiencing them.
- Some patients deliberately don't read the known side effects but they do stay alert when they begin taking a new medication. If they suspect they are experiencing a side effect, they then read what's written and attempt to determine if they are indeed being affected. The next step of course is to notify the doctor. There are so many variations of most known medications that a different version of the same medication may prove to be side-effects free.

Allergic Reactions—Make note of any sensitivity or reaction to the products. Make sure you note the date, time, place, and describe in detail the reaction. It might range from just a feeling of discomfort or headache or stomachache to something as severe as a swollen tongue, severe rash or seizure. Always tell your doctor of any known allergies.

Note: Use two lines if need be to describe your response to the product in detail. Be sure to tell how effective it is, or is not. If discontinued, give the reason.

Medication	Dosage & Frequency	For (Condition)	Prescribing Physician	Date Begun	Date Finished

Remember a log is sequential and ongoing. It answers the fact questions—*who, what, when, where, how* and *why*.

Allergic Reactions—Make note of any sensitivity or reaction to the products. Make sure you note the date, time, place, and describe in detail the reaction. It might range from just a feeling of discomfort or headache or stomachache to something as severe as a swollen tongue, severe rash or seizure. Always tell your doctor of any known allergies.

Over-the Counter Drugs	Dosage & Frequency	For (Condition)	Prescribing Physician	Date Begun	Date Finished

Supplements

Remember a log is sequential and ongoing. It answers the fact
questions—*who, what, when, where, how* and *why.*

As a result of a routine or special need visit to your doctor, you might be asked to have various tests and procedures done, such as x-ray, mammogram, pap smear, EKG, stress test, sigmoidoscopy or colonoscopy and many, many others. The results of these tests and procedures will enable your doctor to evaluate your medical condition and offer medicine, surgery, and/or lifestyle changes, which will improve your health.

> *Note: Summarize all test results on* Chart 2n–Results Log of Screenings, Tests & Procedures *before placing the originals in the Holding Pouch at the back of your notebook.*

Keep Copies It's important that you ask for copies of the doctor's notes and recommendations at the end of each office visit, as well as the results of all tests, and medical procedures—for your own information, as well as to provide a backup of all pertinent information for your healthcare providers. Use the *Health Log (Chart 2b)* to access important information quickly. Be sure to include test results and typed summaries, as well as all of the following:

Adult Immunizations
- Tetanus/Diphtheria
- Pneumococcal vaccine
- Measles/Mumps/Rubella
- Hepatitis *a, b, c*
- Meningococcal
- Chicken Pox
- Lyme vaccine
- Tuberculosis Skin Test

Routine Physical Exams
- General Physical
- Rectal
- Stool Occult Blood
- Pelvic
- Breast
- Prostate
- Dental
- Vision

X-Rays
- Chest X-Ray
- Mammogram
- DEXA Scan
- CAT Scan
- MRI
- Dental
- Bone Density

Doctors Reports
- Office Visit Analysis
- Consultation
- Hospital Discharge Summary
- Eye Exam
- Dental Exam

Heart Testing
- Ekg (electrocardiogram)
- Cardiac Stress Tests
- Cardiac Echogram (ultrasound)
- Cardiac Catheterization
- Ultra Sound

Lab Reports
- Blood Work
- Urinalysis
- Pap Smears
- Biopsies
- Cultures

Screenings and Diagnostic Procedures
- Sigmoidoscopy
- Colonoscopy
- Lung Function Test
- Allergy Test
- Operative Summary
- AIDS
- Hepatitis

2 k   COMMON TESTS RESULTS GRID

This form is designed to help you track test results over time and compare previous tests with current results. This format allows you to trace your medical history quickly, and note your progress. Ask your doctor to set the norms. Using this summary and comparison, you and your doctor can decide if you are on track or if you need to make changes.

Norms	Test	Date Result	Date Result	Date Result	Date Result
	Weight				
	Blood Pressure				
	Heart Rate				
	Hemoglobin A 1c				
	Cholesterol				
	HDL–good				
	LDL–bad				
	Triglycerides				
	Height				
	Bone Density				
	Mammogram				
	Pap Smear				
	Prostate–PSA				

• Listed here are the adult immunizations usually recommended.

• Be sure to update this chart each time an immunization is received.

• It's important to note the date each time an immunization is given or repeated.

• Attach childhood immunization records to this chart.

	Date	Date	Date
Tetanus/Diphtheria (Td) Every 10 years, from age 19	_____ _____	_____ _____	_____ _____
Pneumococcal (pneumonia vaccine) 19-65 if at risk, and at age 65	_____ _____ _____ _____ _____ _____ _____	_____ _____ _____ _____ _____ _____ _____	_____ _____ _____ _____ _____ _____ _____
Measles, Mumps, Rubella (MMR) If vaccination history unreliable	_____	_____	_____
Hepatitis *a* If at risk **Hepatitis *b*** If at risk **Hepatitis *c*** If at risk	_____ _____ _____	_____ _____ _____	_____ _____ _____
Chicken Pox (varicella) If at risk	_____	_____	_____
Influenza Vaccine (flu shot) Age 19-49 if at risk; Annually after age 50	_____ _____ _____ _____ _____ _____ _____	_____ _____ _____ _____ _____ _____ _____	_____ _____ _____ _____ _____ _____ _____

Source: Centers for Disease Control **www.cdc.gov**. *Check with CDC regularly, or your doctor, for changes in recommendations and for immunizations—for malaria, cholera or yellow fever—which might be required to travel to foreign countries.*

Regular checkups and routine exams are necessary to monitor your health and to catch any problem at an early stage. Your doctor, dentist and eye doctor will let you know how often to schedule a check-up and will usually remind you of your upcoming visit.

Doctors use routine screening devices and tests to make sure you're OK. **If something needs medical attention, the sooner it's detected the better**.

Your doctor will already have a test schedule for you in your file in the office. Because you plan to have a good partnership with your doctor, you will want to have a copy of that list so you will know what to expect. Ask for a schedule of any upcoming screenings and exams for your own records. This way you can double check that everything is on target and you won't be taken by surprise.

Age and the overall condition of your health will dictate which of the common tests should be scheduled for you and when. A serious health condition such as cancer, diabetes or heart disease will also affect your particular testing schedule. For these reasons we have not listed every medical test available to physicians, only the most common ones.

Medical Procedures/Exams	**When**
Routine Monitoring	
Physical	As directed by doctor
Height	During routine physical
Weight	During routine physical and/or at every office visit
Blood Pressure	Every office visit; monitor closely if more than 140/90
Heart Rate	Every office visit
Diabetes Tests	
Blood Glucose	45 & older, every 3 years
Hemoglobin A1c	Every 3 months if diagnosed diabetic
Cholesterol	Every 5 years or as directed by doctor
HDL—good	
LDL—bad	
Triglycerides	

(continued on next page)

Common Screenings/Tests	When
Gynecological	
Breast Self-Exam	20 & older: monthly
Clinical Breast Exam	20-39: every 3 years; 40 & older: annually (Sooner if there is a family history.)
Mammogram	40 & older: annually (Sooner if there is a family history.)
Pelvic Exam/Pap Smear	At 18 or onset of sexual activity: annually (Sooner if there is a family history.)
Heart	
EKG	As directed by doctor
Stress Test	As directed by doctor
Cardio-Echogram	As directed by doctor
Colon & Rectal Exams	50 & older

• Fecal Occult Blood Test
  & Flexible Sigmoidoscopy
  with Digital Rectal Exam
	Annually & every 5 years

• Colonoscopy with Digital	Every 10 years
• Rectal Exam	
• Double-Contrast Barium Enema & Digital Rectal Exam	Every 5-10 years
• Rectal Prostate Exam	
Thyroid	As directed by doctor
Bone Density	As directed by doctor
Eye Exam	40: baseline exam; 40-64: every 2-4 yrs. 65 & older: every 1-2 years; diabetics: yearly
Dental Checkup	Every six months
Hearing Test	If hearing problem or loss is suspected

Date_____   **Doctor**_____   **Phone**_____
Condition_____
Test _____
Results_____
Follow-up _____

Date_____   **Doctor**_____   **Phone**_____
Condition_____
Test _____
Results_____
Follow-up _____

Date_____   **Doctor**_____   **Phone**_____
Condition_____
Test _____
Results_____
Follow-up _____

Date_____   **Doctor**_____   **Phone**_____
Condition_____
Test _____
Results_____
Follow-up _____

Date_____   **Doctor**_____   **Phone**_____
Condition_____
Test _____
Results_____
Follow-up _____

Date_____   **Doctor**_____   **Phone**_____
Condition_____
Test _____
Results_____
Follow-up _____

Date_____   **Doctor**_____   **Phone**_____
Condition_____
Test _____
Results_____
Follow-up _____

PART 3
GENERAL HEALTH MAINTENANCE and BASIC MONITORING

Note: Be sure to make copies of all blank charts before using.

Good Eye Care is Preventative in Nature

Wear quality sunglasses, eye protection for hazardous sports, and safety goggles when working with dangerous tools or chemicals. See your eye doctor at the first sign of problems. The four most common and serious threats to vision are:

- Diabetic retinopathy
- Macular Degeneration
- Cataracts
- Glaucoma

Eye Exams

Ask your primary physician how often you should have routine eye examinations.

Use your Eye Care Log to record all eye examinations. Enter all other important information—notes, referrals, treatments, recommendations, results, date of next examination, etc.

Make Specific Note of:

- Prescriptions
- Source of glasses—supplier & manufacturer
- Source of contact lenses—supplier & manufacturer
- Give details of any eye diseases—glaucoma, macular degeneration, cataracts
- Excessive exposure to sun (sunburn)
- Exposure to toxic substances

Eye Injuries

Be sure to describe where and how they occurred, how they were treated and any necessary follow up.

Beware of the Sun

Because the sun is stronger than ever, the best eye care is preventative in nature. Make a habit of wearing sun block and sunglasses. It's very important to train young children to protect themselves from the sun's rays. They need to wear hats, sun block and dark glasses. Remember, if you can see the sun, the sun can see you!

Resource

The Internet address for the American Optometric Association is **www.aoanet.org**.
Use it for additional information relating to the health of your eyes.

3a   EYE CARE LOG

Although you will want to list your primary physician, your ophthalmologist, and your optometrist in your regular address book, for quick reference list them here as well.

Date	Event	Physician/Facility
Rx	Treatment	Results

_____

_____

_____

_____

_____

_____

_____

_____

_____

_____

_____

_____

_____

_____

_____

_____

_____

_____

_____

_____

_____

_____

_____

_____

_____

_____

_____

_____

_____

_____

_____

_____

_____

_____

_____

_____

_____

Remember a log is sequential and ongoing. It answers the fact
questions—*who, what, when, where, how* and *why*.

Hearing loss usually comes on so gradually that others notice the warning signs of hearing loss before you do. Friends and family members are the first to be aware. They can only tolerate your responding, "Excuse me," so many times before they shout, "You need to get your hearing checked!" If they're yelling it, it's probably true.

Warning Signs You Might Also Notice:
- Ringing or buzzing in your ears.
- Sensitivity to loud noises.
- Difficulty hearing others when there is background noise.
- People seem to be mumbling or talking too quickly.
- You always turn up the volume on the TV or radio.
- You hear better with one ear than the other.

Primary physicians always check ears during routine examinations. They might handle a complaint about hearing by simply flushing wax out of the ear. If there is any sign of infection they will usually prescribe an antibiotic.

If there is anything unusual or significant your doctor will likely refer you to an ear, nose and throat specialist or to an audiologist (hearing specialist) who can check the amount of hearing loss and the extent of damage to your hearing.

After analyzing the results of an audiogram (a hearing test which verifies the degree of hearing loss) the audiologist might recommend you to a reputable hearing aid supplier.

Hearing aids are a bit tricky but most people are surprised and relieved at how well they help one hear.

Note: Wear earplugs when you mow the lawn, do target shooting, play video games, or use power tools. Hearing loss due to loud noise exposure cannot be retrieved.

Hearing Aid

By the age of 55, 20% of people have hearing loss. By 65, the number goes up to 33%. Although age-related hearing loss does not typically lead to complete deafness, it does mean one in three people over 65 might do well to consider wearing a hearing aid.

It's Important To Make Note Of All Relevant Information

Date_____

Prescribing practitioner _____

Prescription for hearing aids _____

Device _____

Supplier_____

Manufacturer _____

Remember to record all ear examinations. Include any injuries, how they occurred, and treatments.

Date	Event	Physician/Facility
Rx	Treatment	Results

_____
_____
_____
_____
_____
_____
_____
_____
_____
_____
_____
_____
_____
_____
_____
_____
_____
_____
_____
_____
_____
_____

Remember a log is sequential and ongoing. It answers the fact
questions—*who, what, when, where, how* and *why*.

Tooth Decay

The most common non-contagious disease in the world is tooth decay. It starts with bacteria that live in a sticky film of plaque on the teeth. It feeds off the carbohydrates (sugars) in food, and produces acid in the mouth. The acid erodes the tooth enamel and causes cavities.

Remember the Basics
- Brush for 2-3 minutes morning and night.
- Clean your tongue in the morning to remove bacteria.
- Floss daily, preferably at night.
- See your dentist twice a year for professional cleaning and a cavities checkup.
- Ask the dentist about fluoride treatments for children's teeth.

Avoid high-sugar foods and drinks, especially sticky, sweet foods. The longer sugar stays in touch with your teeth, the more damage it will do.

Foods high in carbohydrates or acid are the worst. Sucking on hard candy or slowly sipping soda or juice all day could be worse than eating a candy bar.

Foods like milk and nuts are *low-risk* foods, not only because they are low in sugar and high in protein, calcium and phosphorous, but because of their non-sticky texture.

Sticky foods put teeth at a greater risk for dental cavities because the food stays in contact with the teeth longer. Grapes and raisins are both healthful fruits, but raisins are more harmful to teeth than grapes because they are stickier and can sneak into tooth crevices.

Better Choices
- Replace sugary foods with fruits, vegetables and high-protein snacks.
- Because fruits and vegetables are also high in water and fiber they lessen the effects of sugar on teeth.
- High-protein foods (milk, nuts, cheese) do not cause tooth decay.
- Tooth healthier snack choices are cheese, raw vegetables, crunchy fruits, popcorn, nuts, and artificially-sweetened beverages.

3c   DENTAL CARE LOG

In this Dental Log keep track of:

- Routine examinations (twice a year)
- Braces
- X Rays

- Fillings, caps, bridges, dentures
- Periodontal problems & treatment
- Surgery

| Date | Event | Physician/Facility |
| Rx | Treatment | Results |

_____

_____

_____

_____

_____

_____

_____

_____

_____

_____

_____

_____

_____

_____

_____

_____

_____

_____

_____

_____

_____

_____

_____

_____

_____

_____

_____

_____

_____

_____

_____

_____

_____

Remember a log is sequential and ongoing. It answers the fact
questions—_who, what, when, where, how_ and _why_.

3d SKIN CARE LOG

In this Skin Care Log keep track of:
- Doctor's Office Visits/Procedures
- Serious skin episodes
- X Rays
- Surgeries
- Allergic Reactions
- Alerts

Date	Event	Physician/Facility
Rx	Treatment	Results

_____
_____
_____
_____
_____
_____
_____
_____
_____
_____
_____
_____
_____
_____
_____
_____
_____
_____
_____
_____
_____
_____
_____
_____
_____
_____
_____
_____
_____
_____
_____
_____

Remember a log is sequential and ongoing. It answers the fact
questions—*who, what, when, where, how* and *why*.

HEALTH AND ACCIDENTS

The one place we spend most of our adult waking lives is at work. It stands to reason that, given the amount of time we spend there, it is likely we will have health or accident related incidents on the job.

Compensation for time lost from the job, for partial or total disability, or actual loss of job, is provided only where there is a clear and factual record.

Work related health issues such as exposure to toxic substances, stress, allergies, accidents, and work related illness, need to be carefully documented. It's important to include all relevant details.

Make Careful Note Of:

Environment
Make note of the occupational hazards of the job, the pressure and pace of the job, the noise level, the presence of chemicals, the number and kinds of accidents, etc.

Safety Awareness
The level of training offered by the company, the emphasis on safety, the monthly and yearly safety record.

Injuries
Broken bones, sprains, strained or pulled muscles, back injuries, cuts, bruises, head injuries.

Delayed Reactions
Because some illnesses and injuries might have complications which show up at a later date, it is important to include all details when incidents first occur.

Ongoing Issues
Make special note of a long series of office visits or an actual hospitalization. It's important to know when they began, the seriousness and when they ended.

Note: Be careful to be precise about the date so that, if asked, your doctor's office will be able to locate their records promptly.

Date   Event   Physician/Facility
Rx   Treatment   Results

_____
_____
_____
_____
_____
_____
_____
_____
_____
_____
_____
_____
_____
_____
_____
_____
_____
_____
_____
_____
_____
_____
_____
_____
_____
_____
_____
_____
_____
_____
_____
_____
_____
_____

Remember a log is sequential and ongoing. It answers the fact
questions—*who, what, when, where, how* and *why*.

A simple listing of where you worked, and when, and what your job assignment was, will provide additional information that will help you keep track of your work related health history.

| Name | Hiring Date | Starting Wage | Starting Responsibility |
| Address | Leaving Date | Leaving Wage | Leaving Responsibility |

_____

_____

_____

_____

_____

_____

_____

_____

_____

_____

_____

_____

_____

_____

_____

_____

_____

_____

_____

_____

_____

_____

_____

_____

_____

_____

_____

_____

_____

_____

_____

_____

Remember a log is sequential and ongoing. It answers the fact
questions—*who, what, when, where, how* and *why.*

FEMALE REPRODUCTIVE HEALTH

It's important to keep your reproductive system healthy—whether or not you plan to have children. Your overall image of yourself as a woman is greatly influenced by your reproductive health, even when you have passed the childbearing years.

Make an effort to learn about your reproductive system so that you can keep it in good working order. The female system is complicated and subtle. So many factors are intertwined, each one impacting on the other.

Describe in your log all relative activity. Be sure to make note of what is going right, as well as your mental state. Irregularities or changes in patterns show up best when compared to normal activity.

Keep careful and detailed track of the following:
- Puberty
- Menstrual cycle, age first period, regularity, difficulties
- Reproductive system
- Sexual activity—age commenced
- Birth control
- Gynecological exams—pap smears, mammograms, etc.
- Hospitalizations
- Pregnancy, pre-natal tests, doctor visits
- Childbirth
- Menopause
- Difficulties—infertility, cancer, sexually transmitted diseases, etc
- New knowledge
- Mental health

Once you have recorded specific information in the Female Reproductive Health Log, be sure to staple together all papers relating to any specific incident, and store them in the *Holding Pouch* in the back of your *Red Notebook*.

Date	Event	Physician/Facility
Rx	Treatment	Results

_____
_____
_____
_____
_____
_____
_____
_____
_____
_____
_____
_____
_____
_____
_____
_____
_____
_____
_____
_____
_____
_____
_____
_____
_____
_____
_____
_____
_____
_____

Remember a log is sequential and ongoing. It answers the fact
questions—_who, what, when, where, how_ and _why._

Our mental/emotional state is the most important aspect of our daily lives. It is the first thing noticed by everyone we live with, work with, and play with.

We feel good mentally and emotionally when we have energy, good health, satisfaction, happiness, warmth, and joy in our lives. We run into trouble when our mental and emotional health begins to be described with words like sad, depressed, anxious, overwhelmed, angry, belligerent, resentful, disoriented, disconnected, and withdrawn.

It's natural to have highs and lows in our day to day activities whether we are alone or in the company of others. However, when an ongoing feeling of things being out of hand becomes our primary mode, we need to seek help from our family, friends, and doctors to get things back on track.

Keeping a log of these various efforts will provide insight and create a history if a more serious concern develops.

Depression Affects Many Older Americans

In formerly mentally healthy individuals, depression can be brought on by loss of a spouse, by divorce, or by illness or being diagnosed with a serious disease. It can be a side effect of certain medications.

Depression is often the cause of sleeping problems, fatigue, or weight loss which might be attributed instead to diabetes or heart disease. One in five Alzheimer's patients suffers from depression.

Fortunately, most people who are depressed respond very well to anti-depressant medications, although sometimes more than one must be tried to find one that is the most effective.

Date	Symptoms	Doctor
Facility	Therapy	Rx
Results	Follow up	

_____
_____
_____
_____
_____
_____
_____
_____
_____
_____
_____
_____
_____
_____
_____
_____
_____
_____
_____
_____
_____
_____
_____
_____
_____
_____
_____
_____
_____
_____
_____
_____
_____
_____
_____
_____

Remember a log is sequential and ongoing. It answers the fact
questions—_who, what, when, where, how_ and _why_.

Each of us, at some point in time, will need some extra help to keep us looking and feeling well.

We will be grateful for the portable oxygen tanks and air filters, as well as the dialysis machines, that give us clean air and clean blood. We will get invaluable help in monitoring, treatment, and prevention from the blood pressure, blood sugar, and heart monitoring machines that enable us to keep track of how we're doing.

It's important to document all medical devices and equipment. You might need to have them repaired or replaced.

In your ongoing medical files keep either the originals or copies of prescriptions, directions, receipts, and the addresses of suppliers—both the retailers and the manufacturers. Be sure to make note of the name and phone number of anyone in the company you have contacted personally.

Date	Medical Aid	Physician
Supplier	Address/Phone	

_____

_____

_____

_____

_____

_____

_____

_____

_____

_____

_____

_____

_____

_____

_____

_____

_____

_____

_____

Remember a log is sequential and ongoing. It answers the fact
questions—*who, what, when, where, how* and *why*.

ALTERNATIVE THERAPIES

Alternative, or complementary therapies, are becoming increasingly popular, with chiropractic, acupuncture, shiatsu, and yoga being some of the better known. More and more people are using alternative therapies to help cope with stress, allergies, diet, and physical problems.

Below Is A List Of Almost 40 Major And Minor Alternative Therapies In Current Use, Often In Conjunction With Orthodox Medical Treatment.

Eastern Therapies: Acupuncture, Auricular Therapy, Shiatsu & Accupressure, Chinese Herbalism, Ayurvedic Medicine, Polarity Therapy

Manipulative Therapies: Osteopathy, Cranial Osteopathy, Chiropractic, Massage, Reflexology, Metamorphic Technique

Natural Therapies: Aromatherapy, Homeopathy, Nutritional Therapy, Western Herbalism, Naturopathy, Bach Flower Remedies

Active Therapies: Relaxation & Visualization, Alexander Technique, Hypnotherapy, Yoga, Tai Chi, Autogenic Training

Therapies Involving External Powers: Spiritual Healing, Color Therapy, Crystal & Gemstone Therapy, Cymatics, Radionics

Bodywork: Rolfing, Hellerwork & Biodynamic Therapy

Arts Therapies: Art Therapy, Dance/Movement Therapy, Music Therapy, Drama Therapy

Diagnostics Therapies: Kinesiology, Iridology, Kirlian Photography

Benefits of Alternative Therapies

Complementary practitioners often take an hour or more to find out about you as opposed to the 15 minutes typical for conventional doctors. Many health concerns are successfully met by the holistic approach more typical of the alternative methods. Complementary treatments often involve careful listening to and touching patients, which is helpful to many people. People who are stressed are more likely to become ill; practices like yoga and tai chi help ease stress and offer calm and serenity. Finally, having access to alternative practices gives many patients/clients a sense of control over their health destiny.

Caution: These therapies range from proven usefulness to the most dubious. Use common sense to choose what's right for you. If you are using one or more of the therapies listed, either short term or ongoing, it's important to keep track of their use and efficacy, and to keep your medical doctor informed.

Resource: For more information about alternative or complementary treatments contact the National Center for Complementary and Alternative Medicine (NCCAM) at the National Institutes of Health: NCCAM Clearinghouse, P.O. Box 8218, Silver Spring, MD 20907-8218 (1-888-644-6226)

3k   ALTERNATIVE THERAPY LOG

Date	Practitioner/Facility	Treatment/Results

Remember a log is sequential and ongoing. It answers the fact
questions—*who, what, when, where, how* and *why*.

PART 4
KEY FITNESS and OVERALL HEALTH

Note: Be sure to make copies of all blank charts before using.

PART 4.1
STRESS MANAGEMENT

Note: Be sure to make copies of all blank charts before using.

The Three Greatest Obstacles To A Healthy Life Are Stress, Inactivity And Overweight.
It is highly unlikely that people who are suffering from chronic stress are able to have any degree of success with either regular exercise or weight loss.

Stress Can Be Both Good and Bad
So long as we are alive and breathing it's impossible to eliminate stress. Stress energizes and motivates us. Stress is not only external (spouse, family, money, job, boss, traffic) it is also our running internal dialogue (our response to our spouse, family, traffic, boss, etc.) Stress not only comes from negative events such as job loss, divorce, illness, or death, but also from happy events like birth, marriage, holidays, parties, and time with friends.

Although some people become violent or abusive in response to stress, many people try to relieve the symptoms of stress by either becoming couch potatoes—lying about gobbling comfort foods—or by smoking, drinking, using drugs, or by just shutting down or being depressed. These efforts at self-medication ultimately leave them dull and exhausted.

Stress can also make some people hyperactive and driven, with no balance in their lives. They become sleep-deprived workaholics. Always grumpy and insensitive, they snap at people and throw tantrums. They have no patience. They create tension in themselves and for other people who describe working with them as a nightmare.

"May the Stress Be With You"
You are handed this little Yoda-type message on the day you are born. "As long as you live, you shall have stress in your life." Will you remember your speech? Will the wedding go O.K.? Will the baby be born healthy? Will you get the job? Can you do the job if you get it? What will be inside the beautifully wrapped box? Will it rain at the picnic? Can we sell the house before we move? Did we ask enough for it? Are we asking too much? Do I look O.K. in this dress? Will his mother like me? Can I finish by 4 o'clock? Will the test come back negative? Where are the kids? What was that noise?

Positive or negative, all changes and challenges—physical, mental, psychological, and social— are stressful to varying degrees.

The most significant thing about stress is that when we respond—with anxiety, tension or worry—that response is not just *mental*. When we feel threatened in any way, chemicals are released, producing physical changes such as rapid pulse rate, quick breathing and dry mouth. These changes prepare the body for *fight or flight*. If we react to stress over long periods of time we experience chronic stress which usually results in some degree of physical or emotional illness.

Because stress impacts so significantly, learning more helpful ways to deal with the symptoms of stress can improve the quality of life tenfold.

Prolonged, Chronic Stress
Most people in today's world, are beset by some very serious and many seemingly trivial

stresses. Fear of terrorism, poor health, concern for our families, our jobs and our homes, crowds, noise, death of a family member, information overload, too many choices, high expectations, power outages, overdue library books, rudeness, parking tickets, equipment breakdowns, holidays, incompetence, traffic, credit cards, vacations, home/cell/work phones, commuting, shoddy workmanship, divorce, stock market fluctuations, single-parent families, email, the Internet, technology, loud music, politics, news, charities, citizenship, celebrities, day care, elder care, shopping, cleaning, maintaining, zero down-time.

No wonder we all liked those Tarzan movies so much. "Me Tarzan, you Jane, him Boy, let's vine up to the escarpment, eat some fruit, curl up in a pile of leaves and take a nap." What a life—Tarzan to keep us safe and Cheeta for comic relief. By the way, what is an escarpment, anyway?

The Bad News
The bad news is stress is here to stay. It's everywhere and it won't go away. As long as we're alive we will face stress with every new event, every surprise, every choice, every challenge.
The Good News is Twofold.
- Stress is easy to identify since we react so instantly.
- There are many effective ways to combat stress.

STRESS TRIGGERS PHYSICAL, MENTAL AND SOCIAL RESPONSES

Physical Response To Stress
We experience acute distress when something out of the ordinary happens—when something big challenges us, such as getting fired or being in a serious accident, or even being crowned Miss America. We respond immediately and physically with a pounding heart, a knot in the stomach, and shallow breathing. We become hyper-alert, disoriented, even hysterical. We might faint. Believe it or not, these responses are exactly right and they actually help us to handle quite well a single event of acute distress.

Fight or Flight
Your body is programmed to respond when under threat. A snarling brown bear suddenly appears in your path as you're hiking the Appalachian Trail. Quick as a finger snap your brain sounds the alarm and sends out stress hormones. Your body flies into instant action. At the first sign of alarm, chemicals released by the pituitary and adrenal glands and the nerve endings automatically trigger physical reactions to stress.

Stored fats and sugar pour into your bloodstream for energy. Your breathing rate increases because you're going to need more oxygen in your blood. Your heart beats faster and your blood pressure increases to carry the extra blood needed to carry that oxygen. The digestive system slows down so the blood normally used to digest food can also be used for the all-important oxygen.

You start to perspire more heavily. Your pupils dilate. Blood-clotting systems are alerted just in case you are injured. You feel a rush of strength. Your body is tense, alert, and ready for action. In the blink of an eye you now stand to fight brown bear—or to take flight.

After this natural alarm reaction to a real or perceived threat, your body stays on alert until you feel that the danger has passed. Then your brain signals an "all clear" to your body, and your body stops producing the chemicals that caused the physical reaction and gradually returns to normal.

Emotional Stress Also Has Physical Consequences

Obviously the *fight or flight* response we've just described is exactly the right thing when faced with a huge physical challenge from brown bear, where our lives are at immediate risk. However, this same set of physical responses isn't so helpful when faced with constant emotional stress. When our bodies react to a traffic backup in the same way it responds to brown bear, it's more harmful than helpful.

Inappropriate Physical Responses Actually Add to the Prolonged and Chronic Stress of Modern Life

Problems with stress occur when your brain fails to give the "all clear" signal. If the alarm state lasts too long, you begin to suffer from the consequences of constant stress. You may find it difficult to see the relationship between stress and physical health problems, because the long-term effects of stress are subtle and slow. However, experts in every area of medicine are discovering links between stress, disease, and poor health.

The Result of Constant Stress
- Most adults say they feel highly stressed.
- 25% suffer sleep deprivation caused by stress.
- Most visits to physicians are stress related.
- Most disease and illness is stress related.
- Stress related depression contributes significantly to increasing rates of suicide.
- On-the-job stress is expensive since it causes absenteeism and increased health insurance costs.
- Reduced productivity and higher employee turnover.

Stress and Heart Disease

Stress significantly increases the risk of heart disease—the # 1 killer in the U.S. Stress directly affects the coronary system. It increases cholesterol, raises blood pressure, increases blood clotting, and inflames and constricts arteries. It contributes to abnormal heart rhythms that can cause instant death.

Stress and Obesity

An equally significant result of stress is obesity. Just as the body makes an immediate demand for extra energy when faced with brown bear, it responds exactly the same way for modern day non-physical stressors. Cortisol is a powerful stress hormone that helps the body get the energy it needs in a crisis. When it is released into the system, the body responds by demanding *fats and sugars*. Continuing stress causes the body to hold onto fat cells as an energy reserve. The resulting weight gain inhibits exercise. The result is overweight, which in itself causes more stress. The vicious cycle continues as the body continues to gain weight.

Recognizing Stress

The signs of stress are classic. You may get a headache, stiff neck, or a nagging backache. You may start to breathe rapidly or get sweaty palms or an upset stomach. You may become irritable and intolerant of even minor disturbances. You may lose your temper more often and yell at your family for no good reason. Your pulse rate may increase and you may feel jumpy or exhausted all the time. You may find it hard to concentrate. When these symptoms appear, it's important to recognize them as signs of stress and to find a way to deal with them. Just knowing why you're feeling the way you do may be the first step in coping with the problem. It is your response to stress, not the stress itself, that affects your health the most.

WARNING SIGNS AND SYMPTOMS OF STRESS

Because chronic stress is so pervasive it is important to be alert to the physical, emotional and behavioral signs of too much stress.

Physical Symptoms
- Ringing in the ears
- Muscular tension
- Neck and back aches
- Numbness or tingling
- Chest pains
- Stomach and intestinal problems
- Irregular menstrual periods
- Skin eruptions and cold sores
- Steady and continuous weight gain
- Headaches, grinding teeth, tight, dry throat, clenched jaws, shortness of breath, pounding heart, high blood pressure, muscle aches, indigestion, constipation/diarrhea, increased perspiration, cold or sweaty hands, fatigue, insomnia, frequent illness

Psychological and Emotional Symptoms
- Loss of self-esteem; a feeling of worthlessness
- Hopelessness, depression, feeling trapped, helpless, feeling of insecurity
- Feelings of fatigue and boredom, unhappiness and sadness
- Feeling of impending danger or doom
- Problems with moodiness, apathy
- Anxiety, irritability
- Slowed thinking, racing thoughts
- Feeling of lack of direction, sadness
- Defensiveness, anger, hypersensitivity

Behavioral Symptoms
- Overeating or loss of appetite
- Poor personal hygiene
- Negativity
- Procrastination
- Avoiding or neglecting responsibility
- Increased use of alcohol or drugs
- Change in religious practices

- Change in family or close relationships
- Too tired to exercise
- Oversleeping or not getting enough sleep

Social Symptoms
- A sense of paranoia;
- Increased sensitivity to criticism
- Being short-tempered
- Tendency to criticize and be argumentative
- Rigid behavior
- Withdrawal or isolation

Symptoms At Work
- Poor job performance
- Difficulty making decisions
- A feeling that there "just aren't enough hours in the day" to get things done
- Trouble meeting deadlines
- Poor memory
- A hard time concentrating or being productive or creative
- Burnout

Often a person under great stress can exhibit many of these warning signs simultaneously. The cruel irony is that the reaction to stress may in itself produce more stress in an ever-escalating spiral. Be sure to talk with your doctor or health professional if you experience more than the occasional sign of being overstressed.

TECHNIQUES TO COMBAT AND RELIEVE STRESS

Plan to Mitigate Stress
Since stress is unavoidable, you need a plan to handle it when it comes your way so it doesn't have such a harmful impact on your life. You can gain more control if you understand the origins of stress and it's effect on the body. It's important to learn a variety of ways to mitigate its harmful effects.

Neutralizing the Effect of Harmful Stress
An overabundance of stress causes disease and slowly kills us. Relaxation skills, proper nutrition, daily exercise, and adequate rest help to neutralize stress. So do laughing, positive thinking, meditation, singing, smiling, music, gardening, and deep rhythmic breathing.

Stress Signals the Brain
Stress originates with the brain. When it perceives a threat it telegraphs a warning to the body which instantly takes over and makes physical preparation. By the time the mind realizes what's happening all systems are go.

If you're going to combat chronic stress you have to think of a way to either
- Prevent the automatic response, especially with repeated stressors, or
- Quickly override this brilliant system once the mind gets alerted.

Because stress happens so frequently and in so many different settings, people who deal well with stress have a complete arsenal of techniques to either prevent stress or to lesson its power. They process and manage their stress by using these techniques to:
- Quiet the mind
- Relax the body

PHYSICAL RESPONSES TO SUDDEN STRESS

Breathing — Ways to Slow the Breath to Reduce Stress
- Slowly breathe in and out, taking a total of five deep breaths before responding to anyone or anything that suddenly stresses you. It's physically impossible to breathe deeply and be tense at the same time.
- Visualize breathing in the good air, breathing out the bad. Breathe in the good air to the place that hurts, imagine it scooping up the hurt and breathe it out.
- Breathe in as you count to yourself, "One, two, three." As you breathe out say, "One, two, three, relax." Feel the tension leave as you breathe out.
- Breathe in as you imagine filling up a little balloon that rests inside you, just below your navel. Once it's full, hold it for a second or two, then let the air out. Fill up the little balloon five or six times and see how much more relaxed you feel. See the balloon in your favorite color.

Relaxing the Muscles to Relieve Stress
In sequence tense and release large muscle groups. Lie down if possible to do this:
- Breathe in
- Hold your breath while you tense your right arm
- Make your fist especially tight
- Count to six
- Release
- Then shake your arm loose.
- Tighten and release in turn your:
- Left arm
- Right leg
- Left leg
- Torso
- Head and face

Finally, tense your entire body all at once, hold, then relax. Take 3 deep breaths in a row. The relaxation response is the opposite of the stress response. It slows your heart rate and slows your breathing. It lowers your blood pressure and helps relieve muscle tension.

MENTAL RESPONSES TO SUDDEN STRESS
Anger makes you tense, clouds your judgment and makes you ineffective in dealing with others, especially children. Vow to remove it from your list of responses.

Count to Ten

Instead of acting on your first impulse—to get mad—count slowly to ten. If you need to, count to 20, or count to ten backwards.

Visualization

Visualize the person you aspire to be. Try to catch yourself being that person and give yourself a big, "Yessss!" See yourself as easy, natural and graceful. Unhurried, relaxed, free and easy, with a smooth brow and a ready smile, always have a word of gratitude or encouragement at hand. Leave people calm and peaceful and glad to have seen you.

Long Term Strategies for Reducing/Preventing Chronic Stress

We all want to feel good about ourselves and our lives. We want to be healthy and happy. We want to avoid becoming frustrated, irritable, ill groomed, angry, sarcastic, argumentative, disagreeable and contrariwise. We truly do not want to become just another victim of stress.

In order to combat chronic stress we must develop a virtual arsenal of effective responses and preventions. In our struggle to balance work and home we must avoid becoming more and more frazzled. It's crucial that we learn to relax and take care of ourselves. We owe it to ourselves and to our families, our friends and our fellow workers to become centered, happy human beings. And somehow we have to do it with grace and clarity, not by adding one more thing on our things-to-do-list.

PHYSICAL STRATEGIES TO COMBAT CHRONIC STRESS

The Basics — Good Health Habits
- Nutritious food.
- Regular exercise helps burn off excess negative energy from stress. A brisk daily walk may be the single best defense against chronic stress.
- Adequate rest and sleep.
- No smoking or drugs, moderate use of alcohol.

Plus
- Beginner's Yoga, T'ai chi.
- Release of tension through massage therapy or acupuncture.
- Muscle tensing and release exercises used throughout the day.
- Doing what you enjoy; having fun—dancing, singing, biking, reading, visiting, etc.

Move the Tension Away

The body responds to stressful thoughts or situations with muscle tension, which can cause pain or discomfort. For immediate relief, walk, dance, climb stairs, bike, any movement is better than none. A 30 minute walk will blow away the cobwebs, lighten your mood, give you renewed energy, and strengthen your heart. If you must watch TV, stand up and walk, march, run in place and stretch out and over and up and under. Tighten and relax one group of muscles at a time.—make a face, clench your fists, punch out your arms, stiffen your legs, tighten your buttocks, stick out your neck. You'll have fun seeing how weird you can be.

Pursue Healthy Pleasures

Give yourself permission to make yourself happy. The good things in life make it easier to deal with the things that aren't so good. If it's been a while since you've indulged yourself in something pleasurable, try this exercise:

- Make a list of 10 (or more) things that give you pleasure.
- Do at least one of the things on your list every day for a week.
- Enjoy and repeat!

Visual Imagery

- Close your eyes and breathe slowly, regularly and deeply.
- Once you are relaxed, imagine you are in a favorite spot, or a place of great beauty.
- As thoughts flow through your mind, notice them, but do not focus on any of them.
- After 5 or 10 minutes, rouse yourself from the state gradually.

Choose Joy

We can't always control what happens to us, but we can control how we react to it.
Joy truly is a choice. Think of the people you know who look nice, who smile and seem to have such a smooth life. Do you really think nothing bad ever happens to them? You have a choice to make. Choose what's best for you.

Take a Break — Get Away

- Schedule private time each week when you actively renew yourself.
- A change is as good as a rest; take a vacation or a long weekend.
- Get yourself ready for fun. Make preparations. List the things you want to do. Plan, schedule, organize, save, research, anticipate—and just do it!
- Create private time and space—to be alone, to think, to dream.
- Consciously screen out and avoid noise, crowds, hyper-activity—all the clamor of life.
- Use ear phones and quieting tapes if you have to.
- Listen to beautiful, not raucous music.

Long Bath —What is it about water? Whatever it is it's wonderful. Pretend the shower is broken, lock the door and enjoy a half hour to yourself.

Massage — Let the pros find the tightness and tension and work them out for you. You're worth the time and cost. It's a better value than a shopping spree.

Let the Light Shine In — Pay attention to how much light there is, at home and at work, especially in winter. Install a UV light in the bathroom so you can turn it on first thing on winter mornings, and start your day with summer sunshine. It truly does fight those mid-winter blues brought on by short, gray-sky days.

Revive the Simple Life — Focus on your spouse and kids, friends, pets, walks, picnics, flowers, water, trees, music, books, talk. We know a couple with three sons who regularly roasted hotdogs in front of the fireplace on Sunday evenings in the winter, complete with marshmallows on a stick. Everybody reviewed the past week, especially their favorite event or accomplishment, and they all talked about what was coming up next week. It sounds a little too sweet? Maybe, but those three boys are all grown up and self-assured. They are bright and funny, and are each other's best friends.

Don't Buy It, Make It—Before Christmas my friend Susan gives to every family in her extended circle—friends, neighbors, co-workers, and church—a half pound of homemade sugared pecans tied with a red ribbon. She and her kids cook them up and wrap them and distribute them personally. They're delicious and eagerly awaited by one and all; it's how we know Christmas is coming. What does she do with the money she saves on presents for all of us? She donates it in the annual Christmas fund sponsored by our local newspaper.

HELP TO MAKE A HEALTHIER WORLD

Radiate Outwards
Become the center of the universe; it's an extraordinary perspective. Do what you can to make your home, your community, and your world a better place. Support a cause that is working to make positive changes. Recycle. Mentor. Tutor. Volunteer. And remember, Peace on Earth begins at home: seek non-violent ways to resolve conflicts at home, at school, at work, and in your community.

Tune Out the Insanity/Inanity—Turn Off the TV
Avoid cultural trash. Protect your children. We always feel better when we aim for the best, not the worst, of what human beings are capable of doing. You wouldn't allow these violent, vulgar, sadistic, sarcastic people in your front door, so don't let them sneak in via the TV. If you can't regulate TV watching, and most people can't, admit defeat and turn it off.

Besides being a time waster, TV is a distortion of American life and news. Instead of watching the news; read it instead. Reading the news takes 5 minutes instead of 30.

Avoid violent, sensational films; horrific pictures are impossible to erase from the mind.

Don't Let Children Watch TV... Period
If you won't turn it off for yourself, then do it for the kids. There's no such thing as appropriate children's TV or videos. A half hour cartoon or video steals a half hour of childhood. You don't want to be an accomplice in this crime. The precious moments and pastimes that make up childhood are what children are not enjoying while they're watching TV and videos.

It's your decision. You're the adult; they are little children in your care. The millions of violent and vulgar images children take in each day will be there for life and will create the major part of their character. Take a look at programs aimed at young children—10-year-olds pretending to be 6-year-olds, either cooing and gooing with a big pink dinosaur, or rug rats whining and using teenage slang and sarcastic putdowns while they manipulate other children shown to be less attractive or less powerful.

If you're using the TV as a baby sitter, take a look at who's doing the job. Would you invite a hooker, a gangster, a stripper, a murderer, a rapist, a stupid bully or a terrorist into your home to baby-sit or entertain your children? That's what's happening when the TV is turned on and children are watching or walking past.

MEDITATION—TECHNIQUES FOR QUIETING THE MIND

- Meditate as you breathe. Use your skill of deep breathing as the basis to meditate. Focus on counting your breaths in groups of four. Count silently as you breathe in and out. In,/out-one; in/out-two; in/out-three; in/out-four/ in/out-one; in/out-two… After each set of four breaths start over—one, two, three, four. If you find yourself counting 14, 15, 16, notice it but don't dwell on it. Just go back to one again.
- Attend to passing thoughts. As distracting thoughts enter your mind, notice them but don't dwell on them. Watch them as they drift out of sight like a summer cloud and continue with your meditation.
- Visualization. Watch an imaginary plant grow; sit comfortably, breathe regularly, focus on the plant for several minutes.

LEARN TO RELAX

Techniques such as guided imagery, meditation, muscle relaxation and relaxed breathing can help you relax. Your goal is to lower your heart rate and blood pressure, slow your breathing and reduce muscle tension.

Sit quietly for several minutes, until you are ready to open your eyes. Notice the difference in your breathing and your pulse rate. The key to this exercise is to remain passive, to let distracting thoughts slip away like waves on the beach.

Imagine the Worst

When faced with the unknown, instead of tensing up and worrying about how to handle every possible scenario, focus on just one—the worst case scenario. What if the worst thing that could happen, did happen? Picture yourself surviving it. Become aware that the worst thing probably won't happen, but even if it did, you could survive. Now you know you could definitely handle whatever happens, since you now know you could handle the worst.

Mindfulness

Pay focused attention as you do a routine task like brushing your teeth, washing dishes, folding clothes, waxing the car. It will help you to become centered, less anxious or irritated.

Practice Silence

Don't utter a word for 10, 20 or 30 minutes. Shhh.

Friends

- Develop friendships with people who make you feel good about yourself and life; avoid people who make you feel bad. Remember, what elevates one of us elevates us all; what degrades one of us degrades us all.
- Talk to people you love and trust. Stress and tension affect your feelings. Talking helps. Telling how you feel gives you new insight—either from just hearing yourself or from their caring responses and interest. Don't worry if you cry. It relieves tension and let's you know just how much some things mean to you.

Getting Organized. Remember, Less Really Is More.

Changing One Thing
- Approach one challenge at a time.
- Resolve to make things better—for yourself and those around you.
- Identify the things you can control and those you can't.
- Ask for extra help if you need it to get things under control.
- As you begin to gain control over one difficult area of your life, you'll realize the next one will be easier.

Practical How-To's
- Set realistic goals and deadlines. Setting goals unrealistically high invites failure.
- Prioritize. Stick with your priorities so you can concentrate on what's most important.
- Be flexible or you'll be overwhelmed before you start.
- Break big jobs into smaller units. No one can write a book in a day.
- Decide what you must do, when you must do those things, and how to schedule enough time to do them. Then arrange other tasks around those must-dos.
- List your tasks. in order of difficulty. Label them A, B or C, in order of importance and difficulty. Writing a report is an A. Paying bills is a B. Organizing your stationery supplies is a C. Don't let yourself do a C until all the B's are done. Don't let yourself do a B until the A's are done.
- Schedule uninterrupted time when you're most productive so you can tackle the A's.
- Interruptions and chaos cause most of our stress at work and at home. Turn off phones, pagers, loud conversations, and TV when you're eating, concentrating or resting. Rely on answering machines but make sure you can't hear them when it's down time.
- Avoid going for perfection. There's no such thing, anyway. Try for doing your best. You'll find it's plenty good enough.

De-Clutter — Take Away 7 Things
- Identify a super-cluttered area. Choose any area you have access to, or are fed up with— any place you use for storage of stuff you work with or collect. For instance, you might start with your sweaters. Pick out the 7 you like the least and put them in a bag for Goodwill. You'll be 7 sweaters lighter and your sweater cupboard will be much less cluttered.
- Next week, re-visit your sweaters. If you still feel over-pullover-ed, chuck out another 7 Leave the sweaters; your work with them is done for now.
- It's time to tackle your next unwitting area—perhaps your bursting-at-the-seams bookshelf. Cull out your least beloved 7 from each shelf, and re-organize the remaining books. You're working towards having 1/3 of each shelf empty. If that didn't happen with the first deletion, you'll probably find yourself already thinking about next week's re-visit to the bookshelf.
- Once you have every nook and cranny down to a size you can keep clean and in order, you are ready for a simple idea that will guarantee that you keep your things in order.
- Vow to make it a rule, that whenever you bring something new into your home, car or work-place, you must remove something. This will cause you to think before you buy a replacement or a new gadget, or accept hand-me-downs or throwaways from family or friends.

- Remember, every space should be 1/3 empty at all times, otherwise you have too much stuff there. If drawers, closets, file drawers, cupboards and shelves are always just 2/3 full it will be easy to find things and you'll also be tempted to put things away rather than just stashing them.
- Before you buy something new or accept a friend's discard, decide what it's going to replace. Be prepared to throw away that current possession before you replace it. No, you can't keep both. That's how you created this cluttered world in the first place.
- Notice how much basic materialism contributes to your clutter and daily hassles. Who needs 30 sweaters anyway?

Simplifying Chores

Modern life is hectic and frantic—cooking, cleaning, clothes, shopping, transportation, children (rooms, schedules, activities), work, volunteering, church, meditation, yoga, exercise, illness, school, jobs, hobbies, sports, media, socializing, vacations, holidays—when you make a list of everything you are responsible for, you realize you need to think clearly to manage it all. You need a plan. Otherwise the weight of it all will crush you.

Think quality not quantity. Look at each task separately, then make a plan to do each routine chore in the smartest, easiest, clearest way possible. Lists, schedules, organizers and the concept of simplification are all tools to keep the myriad parts of your life under control.

Actually, We've Heard The Basics All Our Lives:
- A place for everything; everything in its place.
- Keep only the cooking utensils you actually use.
- Keep things you use daily close at hand, things you use weekly or monthly slightly less accessible.
- Put things you use seasonally or yearly in labeled storage in the attic or garage.
- Choose your favorite 30 recipes and rotate them. You'll quickly learn the recipes and shopping list by heart. If you're in the mood for something new – go ahead and cook it. If it becomes a favorite, replace something on the list of 30.
- Do everyday chores daily; make it a family habit to clean as you go and to tidy up after yourselves. Wash up after dinner not later when food is dried on dishes.
- Before you go to bed—tidy up; hang up clothes, put things away, do a load of wash, and get clothes, lunches, and homework ready for the morning. Make it a family habit to leave the bathroom clean. Make the bed as soon as you get up. Learn to be efficient, but not driven. You're trying to make it easier not add another hassle.
- Get on a schedule. Doing some things at the same time, whether it's daily, weekly, or monthly, means that they actually get done. Getting into a routine that everyone is aware of, saves time and squabbling.
- To do deep cleaning of the house on a simple schedule, simply picture the house as a pizza cut into four pieces. Spend two hours and thoroughly clean one slice of pizza every Saturday.
- List the jobs and let each person choose their own fair share. "I'll do my list later," is not acceptable. One's finished when everyone is finished.

- Delegate and let go. Patiently teaching your spouse and kids how to do chores you've always done is not only fair, it will free you up to do things you've set aside for lack of time or energy.
- Make cleaning fun. Clean to music. Use a buddy system. Hide surprises. Appreciate each person's contribution. Get it done and go have fun.

Just Say No To Things That Are Unimportant And Unsatisfying.

Many people are involved in clubs, committees, and projects that they have little or no interest in or commitment to. Stick with a few activities that are meaningful and let the rest go.

Be Uninformed

Stop trying to keep up. Most news is of no consequence to our lives. We can learn about news that is significant to us in 10 minutes a day reading the paper. An easy way to get weather news is to stick your head outside.

Quiet Time is Quality Time

Be a good model for your family by scheduling regular down time for yourself.
With the input of everyone in the family, agree to a few set hours a week with no TV, telephone, radio, music, or computer interference.

Finances

- Money causes the most stress in families. In a materialistic society like ours the temptations are everywhere—especially on TV.
- It's crucial to get money under control. Keep track so you know how much is coming in and how much is slated to go out, and where.
- Save 10% without fail. Save first, before you pay or buy anything.
- Invest your savings; don't just let them sit there. Once you have 3 months salary in savings, you will think twice before going into debt.
- Impulse buying is the #1 enemy. If you can't pay for it now, it's unlikely you can pay for it later.
- Learn to live with a bit less. Most people are working to pay off or get more stuff. It's smart to do without things that will probably just wind up in a closet anyway. Continuing to do without might just help your family wind up without debt.
- Keep debt to an absolute minimum. Use credit cards only for convenience not to delay payment. Legally credit card interest is as high as 22% a year! That's more than one dollar for every take-home dollar. What a throwaway! Pay the card off every month. That way, the card works for you not the other way around.
- Make a game of "getting it cheaper." Plan and do research before you buy. Buy second hand if you can; actually used things are often better quality once they're spruced up a bit.
- Carefully examine every purchase. Question your shopping list. Do you need a haircut? Can you do your own manicure? Can you learn to cut the kids' hair? Can you groom the dog yourself? Can you alter your own clothes? Libraries were here before mega bookstores.

Develop Your Own Code

Create and articulate your own personal code to live by. Include such things as mutual respect, smiling and greeting other people, being a square shooter, being fair, never lying or cheating, listening—really listening—when others talk, being firm and clear but not unfriendly. When you live by precepts important to you, other people get a fix on your boundaries and values very quickly, and don't step over the line so easily.

Knowledge and Outside Help When Things are Overwhelming

- **Be aware**—Learn to recognize the warning signs of stress.
- **Delegate**—By definition the term "overload" means it's too much. Be wise and get help before you crumple under the weight.
- **Who can help**—See the therapist a friend recommends, or see a counselor at work or at church.
- **See a doctor**—Contact your physician or a mental health professional if stress is out of control or you are unable to function well.

Resources for managing stress can be found in the back of the book.

STRESS REDUCTION / HOURLY LOG
      KEEP TRACK FOR A DAY OR A WEEK

When monitoring your progress think in terms of baby steps. The reason we smile and applaud the baby's first steps is that it is a big deal to begin to walk. And it is a big deal for you when you begin to get your stress under control! Don't ignore the failures but focus on the successes.

6 a.m. _____

7 a.m. _____

8 a.m. _____

9 a.m. _____

10 a.m. _____

11 a.m. _____

12 a.m. _____

1 p.m. _____

2 p.m. _____

3 p.m. _____

4 p.m. _____

5 p.m. _____

6 p.m. _____

7 p.m. _____

8 p.m. _____

9 p.m. _____

10 p.m. _____

11 p.m. _____

12 p.m. _____

1 a.m. _____

2 a.m. _____

3 a.m. _____

4 a.m. _____

5 a.m. _____

Note your efforts, problems, successes, feelings, new ideas, new learnings, etc.
Remember a log is sequential and ongoing. It answers the fact questions: who, what,
when, where, how and why.

Just write down anything relevant to stress—insights, triggers, costs, work or home problems. Stick to the fact questions (*who, what, when, where, how and why*) and you will be amazed at the insight you will gain when you go back a day later and read your notes.

_____

_____

_____

_____

_____

_____

_____

_____

_____

_____

_____

_____

_____

_____

_____

_____

_____

_____

_____

_____

_____

_____

_____

_____

_____

_____

_____

_____

_____

_____

_____

_____

_____

_____

_____

_____

_____

_____

_____

4.1c   STRESS REDUCTION EFFORTS

In this Log keep track of:
- Techniques Mastered
- Exercise
- Meditation

- Teachers, Classes
- Books, Tapes
- Breathing

- Better Organization
- Focus
- Successes

Date	Stress Event	Physician/Facility
New Skill	Practice	Results

_____

_____

_____

_____

_____

_____

_____

_____

_____

_____

_____

_____

_____

_____

_____

_____

_____

_____

_____

_____

_____

_____

_____

_____

_____

_____

_____

_____

_____

_____

_____

Remember a log is sequential and ongoing. It answers the fact
questions—*who, what, when, where, how* and *why.*

PART 4.2
EXERCISE
SECOND KEY TO FITNESS and
OVERALL HEALTH

Note: Be sure to make copies of all blank charts before using.

Good health is evidenced by fitness, energy, and enthusiasm. Reduced stress, daily exercise, and a healthy weight are the three magic components. In this section we will focus on daily exercise.

Daily Exercise is the Key

Remember when moving your body with abandonment was fun? It can be again. Here's where you get to play to your heart's content. You can run, you can skip, you can hop. You can dance. You can join a gym and put on fancy exercise togs. You can don a bathing suit, hop into a pool where no one knows you, and bob around like a porpoise—just like you did when you were a kid. You can take a brisk walk outside and remember what the seasons are all about. If you can afford it you can even splurge for a personal trainer—for your health's sake. You can reward yourself with a massage because it's good for you. You can come back to life.

You will feel better, be fitter, and be stronger in the fight against heart disease and high blood pressure, diabetes and even some cancers. You will be more alert and sleep better. You will become more flexible. You will be more efficient and focused. And you will feel so much better about yourself.

Laura's Advice

- It's never too late to start. Any exercise is better than just sitting.
- Start slowly.
- Plan carefully.
- Do something you like. If you enjoy it, you'll be more likely to stick with it.
- Pick a time of day that works best for you. If it stops working for you, find a better time.
- Think about what motivates you? Is it how you look in the mirror? Your health?
  Could it be a reward—such as a manicure or a night out?
- Join forces—with a friend, a class, a gym.
- Keep track on a daily basis.
- Re-evaluate weekly and adjust your plan as needed.
- Celebrate your successes; learn from your missteps.
- Use available resources—TV exercise programs or tapes from the library, a nearby gym or a private trainer.
- Keep it simple at first—a daily walk, daily stretching, weight training 2-3 times a week.
- Add more challenges as you go along—more time, more repetitions, more weights.
- Check with your doctor if you are over 50 and haven't been exercising.
- Ask your doctor for help modifying your exercise program if you have special needs.

FINDING OUT WHAT IT MEANS TO BE FIT

You're fit:

- If you can complete the workday comfortably and have enough energy left over to enjoy the evening.
- If you can walk a mile or so, climb stairs, carry groceries, or run for the bus without being winded, or feeling it in your legs.
- If you can keep up a conversation while taking a brisk walk.

You're not fit:
- If you can't do most of the above.
- If you sit down all day and stay at your desk during lunch then go home to watch TV.
- If you can't keep up with people your age.
- If you avoid walking, climbing or other physical activity.
- If you become out of breath or tired when walking only a short distance.
- If you look tired and dragged out and have lost your sense of fun.

The Positive Effects of Exercise

Regular exercise reduces by 70% the risk of death from the two leading killers—heart disease and cancer.

• Heart:	Pumps more blood with less effort, decreasing your resting heart rate.
• Cholesterol	Improves all cholesterol indicators including HDL and LDL.
• Blood Pressure	Prevents and lowers high blood pressure and hypertension.
• Diabetes	Lowers high blood sugar and helps prevent adult-onset diabetes.
• Bones	Helps avoid osteoporosis.
• Stress	Relieves stress, helps you to sleep better, improves concentration.
• Self Esteem	You look better and your overall sense of self improves.

The Negative Effects of Not Exercising

We are a sedentary nation and each day we become fatter and fatter. We sit at the table and we sit at the computer. We play video games and we watch sports on TV, but only one in four of us exercises regularly. More that 60% of Americans are overweight. The rates of diabetes and cardiovascular disease are soaring. Research shows that African-Americans are disproportionately affected by hypertension, heart disease, glaucoma, diabetes, stroke, and breast and prostate cancers. More and more children are being diagnosed with obesity, heart disease and type 2 diabetes. Inactivity is epidemic throughout our culture.

THE THREE MAJOR TYPES OF EXERCISE

Optimal results are obtained by a mix of exercises:
1. **Aerobic Exercise** will get your heart and breathing rates up and build up your endurance.
2. **Weight Lifting and Resistance** workouts will result in greater strength and a well-toned body.
3. **Flexibility** comes from gentle stretching.

1. Aerobic Exercise Builds Endurance

Aerobic refers to the oxygen needed and supplied by the body when you are engaged in aerobic exercises. Aerobic exercise is any sustained movement that significantly increases your heartbeat and breathing rates. Most experts suggest continuous movement for 30-40 minutes 3-4 days a week. Breathing and exercising steadily sends an increased level of oxygen to your circulatory system. This kind of activity works your heart and your lungs, and it burns up fat.

Note: The best workout raises the heart rate to a target range and keeps it there for at least 20 minutes.

Your target range is 70% of your maximum heart rate (MHR). This is found by subtracting your age from 220. If you are fifty years old you can find your target number easily:

220 - 50=170   70% X 170=119 Thus 119 is your target heart rate for aerobic exercise.

1000 steps a day is becoming a popular daily exercise. Pedometers are an inexpensive way to get immediate feedback. Clip one on your pocket or belt and you can know instantly how close you are to your goal of 1000 steps a day

Aerobic exercise is the ideal way to get your heart rate up and to just get moving—so take a walk—today!

You'll know when you're exerting enough effort. You have reached your target range when you've worked up a sweat (but are not feeling pain). A good rule of thumb is, if you can sing you're not there yet, but you should be able to complete a sentence.

Walking, running, biking, jogging and swimming are the most familiar aerobic exercises. They involve continuously moving large muscle groups such as your leg muscles. Raking leaves, cross-country skiing and dog-walking are more aerobic exercises that vary the routine and keep you moving.

2. Strength Training

Strength training is also called weight training, body toning, body shaping, or body sculpting. It involves resistance to challenge your muscles and can take different forms. Sit-ups, push-ups, kick boxing, crunches, lunges and squats are excellent. Lifting weights is a key component. Most people either lift free weights or more usual, use weight machines. Elastic bands also work well. They involve looping the bands around your hands or feet and pulling against them. Some of these exercises can be done at home with minimal equipment. However, the most efficient way to achieve the positive effects of strength training appears to be using the weight machines in a gym or health club.

Lifting weights challenges your muscles to become firmer and stronger and must be started slowly and monitored carefully. This is *anaerobic exercise* which means to exercise without oxygen. The energy burned by weight lifting produces lactic acid that builds up in the muscles and causes pain. Be sure a knowledgeable person starts you on the weights and approves of any additional weights, since it is easy to hurt yourself by going too heavy too fast. It's especially important to be guided by a professional if you have any physical condition that could be worsened by inappropriate weight lifting.

Strength training on non-consecutive days, two to three times a week for 30 minutes is all that is needed. You'll see results in as few as six weeks.

If you want to stay trim and close to a healthy weight, muscle is the key. Lean muscle tissue is much better at burning calories than fatty tissue is. Even light weight lifting will give you more energy and cause your clothes to fit better. It will lower your blood pressure and help you feel better overall.

3. Stretching for Flexibility and Grace

Gentle stretching is an essential part of physical fitness. The key to safe stretching is to move slowly and gently. Think of grace not power when stretching. Stretch only until you feel a *pleasant pull*, never pain. Always aim for a comfortable and sustained stretch without straining. Think of cats.

Stretching improves range of motion and balance. It maintains the suppleness of muscles, joints and connective tissue. It adds to your fitness routines by making it easier and safer to move. It also decreases stress by releasing muscle tension. Remember, it's essential to warm up by walking or stepping before you do your gentle stretching routines.

Gyms, health clubs and YMC/HA's offer ballet, yoga and T'ai Chi which are gentle stretching exercises that are a pleasure to do. These ways of stretching also help us to become relaxed, centered and positive. These exercises can also be enjoyed at home through tapes. When stretching is done correctly it is very gentle on the body and can be done every day. Many people who meditate do simple stretching yoga exercise prior to their meditation. Warning— straining or strenuous stretching is always harmful.

BEFORE YOU START A FITNESS PROGRAM CHECK OUT YOUR HEALTH

It's risky to start out too enthusiastically by doing too much and being too energetic after having been too inactive. Talk to your health care provider first if you:
- Smoke.
- Are overweight.
- Are more than 40 years old and haven't exercised regularly for a while.
- Have a serious or chronic health condition such as heart disease, diabetes, high blood pressure, lung disease, or kidney disease.

Then Start Smart
- Get your doctor's O.K.
- Easy does it. Don't set yourself up for failure. Don't overdo it.
- Watch out for red flags—nausea, dizziness, extreme shortness of breath.
- Set achievable goals. Exercise often and regularly.
- On a daily basis fit in 30-40 minutes of brisk aerobic exercise.
- Three times a week add in weight-lifting.
- Use the outdoors whenever you can.
- Do what you like. This isn't a bitter pill we're planning on taking here. It's a choice for life so make sure it involves doing what's enjoyable and accessible. Keep it simple so it doesn't require too much "stuff." If you can barely tolerate it in the beginning, you'll wind up not doing it at all.

Exercise Program and Stress Management / Precursors to Diet Program
We suggest you get your exercise plan solidly under your belt before beginning a serious dieting effort. Exercising successfully for three weeks (21 days makes it a habit) will serve as a foundation for the next challenge. Because you will be feeling so much better, more positive and proud of your recent success, you'll be stoked for the more difficult step of correcting your eating habits and losing weight.

Plan for Built-In Success / Check Out the Gyms

Joining a nearby, no-frills gym will give you access to a treadmill or bike as well as weights, at the least cost. Go first as a guest, or ask for a trial membership. You want to choose a place you'll be comfortable going to on a regular basis. Ask your friends and neighbors where the best deals are. Visit and check it out.

The Best Plans Include
- Daily activity.
- Stating up front the amount of time that will be involved.
- A conscious decision as to the degree of exertion involved.

We don't like **choices** like *go for a walk 3 or 4 times a week*, because of that little word *or* it's too easy to put off your walk until **tomorrow**. Have a specific **daily** commitment and pledge to make it if you possibly can. If you miss, you miss. Pay attention to why you missed and try to avoid repeating it. Learn from it but don't beat up on yourself.

A Typical Successful Schedule for Beginners

Sunday	30-40 minute brisk walk
Monday	20-30 minutes of weights, 30 minutes on the treadmill at the gym
Tuesday	30-40 minute brisk walk, stretching program
Wednesday	20-30 minutes of weights, 30 minutes on the treadmill at the gym
Thursday	30-40 minute brisk walk, stretching program
Friday	30-40 minute brisk walk, 30 minutes on the treadmill at the gym
Saturday	20-30 minutes of weights,

LAURA SAYS: Warm Up, Cool Down / Before and After All Exercise Sessions
- Warming up consists of doing at a slower pace the exercise you're planning to do vigorously. Thus walking is a warm up for jogging; trotting is a warm-up for running. If you're going to play golf, take some easy practice swings using the same muscles you'll use for 18 holes.
- Warm ups protect you against injuries and muscle soreness. They prepare the body for the demands of the exercise.
- Shorten your aerobic/strength training sessions if time is short, but don't skip the warm ups or cool downs.
- Slow walking, easy biking, marching in place, etc. are all great warm ups
- Warm ups should take at least 10 minutes.

Exercise Shoes make it easier to work out as well as safer but you need to keep an eye on them. If you have pain in your feet, heels or legs or if you have tendonitis, blisters or calluses, your shoes need to be replaced. Carefully choose your shoes and make sure they fit. Cushioned socks are important also. Make sure you change your socks after each exercise session.

Note: Warm up by stretching to loosen tight muscles. Cool down by shaking out, walking around for five minutes, and then stretching for flexibility. Do a 10 minute warm up walk. The first two weeks choose a pre-aerobic activity (strolling, walking up a short flight of stairs, gardening, dancing) and focus on doing them for a full 20-30 minutes a day, 3 to 5 times the first two weeks. Remember to do cool downs. You're working to establish habits here.

By the third week focus on getting up to your target heart rate and maintaining it for 20 minutes by walking and/or walking up stairs. Add five minutes a day each week until you reach 60 minutes (this will take 8 to 10 weeks).

As you move more and more each week you will increase you endurance and stamina. To keep up your target heart rate, pick up the pace or add inclines.

As you exercise more, read more, and talk to other people who are working out with you, you will become more knowledgeable and more motivated. You will realize the natural progression to a more active aerobic workout is to add more challenging activity while maintaining your regular time schedule. You will eventually be thinking not in terms of simple walking or swimming, but about adding jogging, cycling, inclined walking, etc., to your menu.

Remember muscle doesn't replace fat when you become more active. A winning combination comes into play. Aerobic exercise burns fat; weights/resistance training increases muscle. The net result is you will become leaner (as well and stronger and more fit). You'll soon see the difference in your mirror.

Resources for Fitness and Exercise can be found at the back of the book.

4.2 A   SUGGESTED WEEKLY EXERCISE SCHEDULE

Note: Warm up and cool down by walking for 10 minutes before and after you do aerobic exercise or strength training.

Aerobic Exercise - 20-45 minutes per session

Sunday	Monday	Tuesday	Wednesday	Thursday	Friday	Saturday
Aerobic	Aerobic	Aerobic	Aerobic	Aerobic	Aerobic	Aerobic
Exercise	Exericse	Exercise	Exercise	Exercise	Exercise	Exercise
____ min	____ min	____ min	____ min	____ min	____ min	____ min

Strength Training — Start with 8-12 Reps and work up.

Monday	Wednesday	Friday
Strength	Strength	Strength
Training	Training	Training
—— Reps	—— Reps	—— Reps

Stretching (Ballet, yoga, T'ai Chi, etc.)

Tuesday	Thursday

- **Aerobic Activity** means 20 or more minutes of sustained moving at your target heart rate—70% of (220 minus your age). Walking, climbing, running, jogging, swimming, stepping, cross country skiing, dog walking—these are all aerobic activities.

- **Strength Training** includes lifting free weights and using weight machines and/or exercise bands.

- **Flexibility Training** includes gentle stretching, yoga, T'ai Chi, dance, etc.

Enter your exercise program into your daily planner at the specific time allocated.

Remember—an appointment with yourself is as important as any of your other scheduled meetings.

Notes:

This record will give you a quick overview of how your exercise program is working.
- Gradually increase the amount of time you spend and increase the degree of difficulty.
- The information recorded here will help you make needed adjustments to your routine—such as changing to a better time of day for a specific activity.
- At a glance you will be able to track your success and reward yourself accordingly.
- Note the physical activity and the time. Be sure to include all aerobic and strength training sessions.

EXERCISE

Week 1

Type (time/amt)	Sun	Mon	Tues	Wed	Thurs	Fri	Sat
Walking							
Aerobics							
Strength Training							
Stretching							

Week 2

Type (time/amt)

Walking
Aerobics
Strength Training
Stretching

Week 3

Type (time/amt)

Walking
Aerobics
Strength Training
Stretching

Week 4

Type (time/amt)

Walking
Aerobics
Strength Training
Stretching

Week 5

Type (time/amt)

Walking
Aerobics
Strength Training
Stretching

PART 4.3
WEIGHT MANAGEMENT

Note: Be sure to make copies of all blank charts before using.

People Usually Become Focused On Returning To Their Ideal Weight When They
- No longer feel attractive due to overweight.
- Find their weight interferes with their effectiveness at work and at play.
- Become worried about the well-publicized health risks of overweight.

People Are Eating More And They Are Less Active And More Stressed
Our ancestors were fit. When food was scarce they had to be extremely active just to survive. For the 65% of Americans who are overweight or obese today, losing weight requires a basic change in thinking—a true paradigm shift.

Multiple Causes for Excess Weight
- **Imbalance of fuel**: Weight gain occurs when more calories are taken in than are expended through exercise. Since early man, our bodies have always been very efficient at storing the excess to use when needed. If the storeroom gets too full, we get too fat.
- **Environmental factors**: General affluence as well as family and cultural influences, such as oversize portions and high calorie foods.
- **Increased stress**: Increased eating to relieve anxiety.
- **Media**: Advertising which constantly tempts us to eat when we're not hungry.
- **Huge portions**: Fast food sellers and restaurants in general are offering larger portions because it does not cost them more to do so and it gives a false impression of hospitality and plenty. The end result, of course, is more calories—more fat and more carbs that are the chief culprits for obesity.
- **Availability**: 24 hours a day—at home, at work, at play.
- **Sedentary lifestyle**: We drive everywhere and watch TV for hours (while we snack); we are much less active than our parents and grandparents, let alone our original forbears.
- **Genetics**: A low metabolism rate and/or a family predisposition to overweight. This condition applies to a very low percentage of overweight people.

Calories
- A calorie is a unit used to measure energy—both energy supplied by food and energy created by movement. Your weight stays the same when you use up the same number of calories that you eat.
- The average adult American needs between 1800 and 2200 calories a day to maintain a healthy weight.
- If you habitually eat more than you burn off, you will gain weight over time by storing the extra calories as fat in special cells your body keeps handy.
- If you eat less than you burn off, your body will go to the storeroom where your fat cells are kept and use up some of them.
- *Note: our local paper in March, 2004, reported a 22% increase in the number of calories consumed by the average American woman since 1971, verses a 7% increase by the average American man.*

To Lose Weight and Keep it Off, Establish Short Term and Long Term Goals
There is a generally accepted truism: if you keep doing what you're doing, you'll keep getting what you're getting. To reach your goal of ideal weight, and your follow-up goal of lifetime

weight control, it is absolutely necessary to change. It requires a paradigm shift—a basic change in thinking—a change in your lifelong pattern of eating, exercising and controlling stress.

Changes in thinking involve:
Increased awareness.
New learnings.
Emotional changes in feelings, attitudes, thoughts and beliefs about food.

Behavioral changes in daily habits:
Stress management—learning how to relax and neutralize stress.
Exercise in some way, every day.
Eating well for life.

Being Overweight Puts You at Risk
- High blood pressure
- Heart Disease
- Stroke
- Diabetes
- Certain cancers
- Deteriorating joints
- Chronic back problems
- Gallstones
- Respiratory Problems

Consult your Primary Physician
Before you go on a diet or start an exercise program, inform your primary physician of your plans. If you've been ill or have been totally sedentary for a long while, be sure to get a complete physical before starting. When you get the go-ahead, start off slowly. It's difficult to be patient once you've decided to really bite the bullet and go for it, but remember your body didn't get in this shape overnight. Don't put it into shock by sprinting out of the gate.

Other Professionals Who Can Be of Help
- Registered dietitians for weight control or nutrition counseling.
- Group weight control programs like Weight Watchers or Over-eaters Anonymous.
- Gyms and YW/MCAs have a wide range of exercise and yoga programs.

Many Experts Recommend
A goal of losing 1 to 2 pounds a week requires a decrease of 500-1000 calories per day.
Safe weight loss = long-term weight loss.

Staying Motivated
The only difference between those who succeed and those who don't is persistence.
If you never give up, you will reach your goal. If you keep taking action and make positive attempts you will succeed.

If the goal is to feel better, look better, improve self esteem, have more energy and health for however long you live, then **the journey**—proper diet and exercise— becomes part of your life and you are guaranteed success.

As you travel towards your goal, taking note of but not dwelling on your failures, keeping track of and celebrating all your successes, you will become aware of a simple truth—**it is the journey that counts, not the destination**.

When you take charge of your body, you take charge of your life and your well being.

So—it's time to wake up and take charge.

4.3a   BODY MASS INDEX (BMI)

Before you embark on a serious weight loss effort, it's important to assess your current state of health in relation to your weight. It is generally healthier to have a high percentage of lean muscle mass and a low percentage of body fat. The most useful way of identifying your ideal weight is by calculating your Body Mass Index. Additional information can be had from Chart 4.3b—*Chart of Healthy Weights by Age.*

One way to calculate your body mass index (BMI) is to use skin fold calipers. This is often done for you when you join a gym or weight loss program. You can also calculate your own BMI by using a simple formula: ***weight ÷ (height x height) x 704.5 = BMI.***

An easier way to identify your BMI is to use the following table: **go down** to find your height, and then **go across** to find your weight, then **go up** to find your BMI.

TABLE OF BODY MASS INDEX

BMI Height	19 Weight	20	21	22	23	24	25	26	27	28	29	30	35	40
4'10"	91	96	100	105	110	115	119	124	129	134	138	143	167	191
4'11"	94	99	104	109	114	119	124	128	133	138	143	148	173	198
5'0"	97	102	107	112	118	123	128	133	138	143	148	153	179	204
5'1"	100	106	111	116	122	127	132	137	143	148	153	158	185	211
5'2"	104	109	115	120	126	131	136	142	147	153	158	164	191	218
5'3"	107	113	118	124	130	135	141	146	152	158	163	169	197	225
5'4"	110	116	122	128	134	140	145	151	157	163	169	174	204	232
5'5"	114	120	126	132	138	144	150	156	162	168	174	180	210	240
5'6"	118	124	130	136	142	148	155	161	167	173	179	186	216	247
5'7"	121	127	134	140	146	153	159	166	172	178	185	191	223	255
5'8"	125	131	138	144	151	158	164	171	177	184	190	197	230	262
5'9"	128	135	142	149	155	162	169	176	182	189	196	203	236	270
5'10"	132	139	146	153	160	167	174	181	188	195	202	207	243	278
5'11"	136	143	150	157	165	172	179	186	193	200	208	215	250	286
6'0"	140	147	154	162	169	177	184	191	199	206	213	221	258	294
6'1	144	151	159	166	174	182	189	197	204	212	219	227	265	302
6'2"	148	155	163	171	179	186	194	202	210	218	225	233	272	311
6'3"	152	160	168	176	184	192	200	208	216	224	232	240	279	319
6'4"	156	164	172	180	189	197	205	213	221	230	238	246	287	328

Obesity, Large Waist, and Apple Shape Increase Health Risks.

A BMI of 30 and above, with a waist measurement greater than 40 inches if you are a man or 35 inches if you are a woman, puts you at greater risk for serious obesity-related problems.

Where you "carry" your fat is a significant factor. If you are apple shaped (fat mainly around your waist), you are more likely to develop health problems than if you are pear shaped (fat mainly in your hips and thighs). This is true even if your BMI falls within the normal range.

Losing as little as 5-10 percent of your body weight can lower your blood pressure and reduce other health risks such as heart disease and stroke, and improve your blood sugar levels if you are diabetic.

4.3b   CHART OF HEALTHY WEIGHTS BY AGE

We usually know if we're overweight, but looking at the chart of healthy weight below you can check to see if you're within the suggested guidelines for a healthy weight.

If you do need to lose weight, the formula is simple: eat fewer calories and exercise more and the excess weight will come off.

Remember—extreme dieting *works against* attaining a healthy weight. If your body feels you are starving yourself, it will slow down your metabolism, causing you to conserve fat rather than lose it.

After a week or ten days, check your program to make sure you're losing from 1 to 1.5 pounds a week, and you will find you can more easily keep it off in the long run.

Age-Adapted Healthy Weights for Men and Women
Source: National Institutes of Health

Age Height	20-29	30-39	40-49	50-59	60-69
4'10"	84-111	92-119	99-127	107-135	115-142
4'11"	87-115	95-123	103-131	111-139	119-147
5'0"	90-119	98-127	106-135	114-143	123-152
5'1"	93-123	101-131	110-140	118-148	127-157
5'2"	96-127	105-136	113-144	122-153	131-163
5'3"	99-131	108-140	117-149	126-158	135-168
5'4"	102-135	112-145	121-154	130-163	140-173
5'5"	106-140	115-149	125-159	134-168	144-179
5'6"	109-144	119-154	129-164	138-174	148-184
5'7"	112-148	122-159	133-169	143-179	153-190
5'8"	116-153	126-163	137-174	147-184	158-196
5'9"	119-157	130-168	141-179	151-190	162-201
5'10"	122-162	134-173	145-184	156-195	167-207
5'11"	126-167	137-178	149-190	160-201	172-213
6'0"	129-171	141-183	153-195	165-207	177-219
6'1"	133-176	145-188	157-200	169-213	182-225
6'2"	137-181	149-194	162-206	174-219	187-232
6'3"	141-186	153-199	166-212	179-225	192-238
6'4"	144-191	157-205	171-218	184-231	197-244

(Get Healthy Enough To Go On A Diet After Only 5 Weeks)

+	= Add to your routine
-	= Delete from your routine

WEEK 1	+	Vitamins
WEEK 2	+	Meditation
WEEK 3	+	Walking 45 minutes a day
WEEK 4	+	Eight 8 oz. Glasses of water a day
WEEK 5	-	White powders (salt, sugar, bleached flour)
WEEK 6	+	Yoga
WEEK 7	+	Four small meals a day (instead of three); 500 calories each.
WEEK 8	+	Five small meals a day (instead of four); 400 calories each.
WEEK 9	+	six small meals a day (instead of five); 300 calories each.
WEEK 10	-	Caffeine
WEEK 11	-	Eating after 8 p.m.
WEEK 12	-	Cigarettes

At the end of 12 weeks the first 10 items on this list will be habitual. You will be feeling 100% better and you will be more rested and focused. (And you will have lost some 5-15 pounds.) You will have established a healthy base for continuing these healthful habits and additional good behaviors like more:

Exercise	*Stretching*	*Meditation*	*Varied Cuisine*
Becoming Clothes	*New Friends,*	*Fun & Playing*	*Saying Yes*

4.3d ANALYZE YOU BEFORE YOU START

You already know more than you might realize about how you operate, what brings you success in other areas of your life and what personal qualities you have to keep an eye on if you want to be sure you do a good job. Use that knowledge to prepare yourself for what will ultimately be a successful campaign to increase your health and happiness.

STRENGTHS—Build on these; add more in.

WEAKNESSES — Identify and notice these. As your strengths begin to grow bigger they will eventually crowd out your weaknesses.

4.3e   A SOLID WEEK OF GOALS

STARTING DATE: _____

What Should I Accomplish This Week? Make note of your successes on the last line for each day.

SUNDAY

_____
_____
_____
_____

MONDAY

_____
_____
_____
_____

TUESDAY

_____
_____
_____
_____

WEDNESDAY

_____
_____
_____
_____

THURSDAY

_____
_____
_____
_____

FRIDAY

_____
_____
_____
_____

SATURDAY

_____
_____
_____
_____

DIARY

Use this diary primarily for tracking your dieting efforts but comment on any other contributing activities such as exercise or meditation.

Jot down any insights or overheard words of wisdom.

Make note on Sunday of your weight and your progress for the past week.

Outline your goals for the coming week.

Highlight your daily successes and any particularly healthful/delicious meals.

Notice when you are on target and think why that is. Notice when it's difficult and try to figure out why so you can correct it.

Anticipate upcoming obstacles and write down your planned solutions so you don't get caught up short.

If there is a major problem, take the time to analyze it carefully so you can prevent it next time.

Keep tabs on your successes in all areas of your life. The more plusses you point out to yourself, the more positive and can-do you will become.

Notice the failures, analyze them, but don't beat up on yourself—absolutely no negative self-talk allowed.

Mention any major changes in your life, including changes of medications.

Be sure to tell why you think anything new worked, or didn't.
Do three pluses and a suggestion at the end of each day. Three things you do very well and intend to keep doing. One thing you plan to work to improve.

Plus _____

Plus _____

Plus _____

Suggestion _____

Tell yourself a joke.

STRESS MANAGEMENT   **DIET DIARY**

_____   _____
_____   _____
_____   _____
_____   _____
_____   _____
_____   _____
_____   _____
_____   _____
_____   _____
_____   _____
_____   _____
_____   _____
_____   _____
_____   _____
_____   _____
_____   _____

PHYSICAL ACTIVITY   _____

_____   _____
_____   _____
_____   _____
_____   _____
_____   _____
_____   _____
_____   _____
_____   _____
_____   _____
_____   _____
_____   _____
_____   _____
_____   _____
_____   _____
_____   _____
_____   _____
_____   _____

4.3g   POSSIBLE MEALS (Think out of the box.):

Make a list to have handy when you're planning and shopping.

BREAKFASTS
1 _____
2 _____
3 _____
4 _____
5 _____
6 _____
7 _____
8 _____
9 _____

LUNCHES
1 _____
2 _____
3 _____
4 _____
5 _____
6 _____
7 _____
8 _____
9 _____

CARRY ALONG FOODS
1 _____
2 _____
3 _____
4 _____
5 _____
6 _____
7 _____
8 _____
9 _____

AM SNACK
1 _____
2 _____
3 _____
4 _____
5 _____
6 _____
7 _____
8 _____
9 _____

AFTERNOON SNACK
1 _____
2 _____
3 _____
4 _____
5 _____
6 _____
7 _____
8 _____
9 _____

MORE IDEAS
1 _____
2 _____
3 _____
4 _____
5 _____
6 _____
7 _____
8 _____
9 _____

DINNER
1 _____
2 _____
3 _____
4 _____
5 _____
6 _____
7 _____
8 _____
9 _____

BEFORE BED SNACK
1 _____
2 _____
3 _____
4 _____
5 _____
6 _____
7 _____
8 _____
9 _____

MORE IDEAS
1 _____
2 _____
3 _____
4 _____
5 _____
6 _____
7 _____
8 _____
9 _____

Notes:

4.3h TRY A WEEK OF SIX SMALL MEALS A DAY
300 CALORIES EACH

DATE _____

	Sun	Mon	Tues	Wed	Thurs	Fri	Sat
7-8 a.m. Breakfast							
10-11 a.m. Snack							
12-1 p.m. Lunch							
3-4 p.m. Snack							
6-7 p.m. Dinner							
8-9 p.m. Before Bed Snack							

Notes:

4.3i   DETAILED DAILY CHART OF SIX SMALL MEALS

DATE _____   **YESTERDAY'S TOTAL CALORIES** _____

	Amount Food	**Fat** (Saturated)	**Fat**	**Carbs**	**Calories**	**Comments**
Breakfast						
Snack						
Lunch						
Snack						
Dinner						
Snack						

Today's Total Calories: _____

4.3j   WEIGH YOURSELF DAILY OR WEEKLY

Watch the numbers go tumbling down.

DATE	DAILY or WEEKLY	DATE	DAILY or WEEKLY

4.3k WEIGHT LOSS LOG

_____ Name
_____ Date
_____ Ideal weight
_____ Rate of weekly loss to reach my ideal weight
_____ Target date to reach my ideal weight

Weight Chart

Date	Weight	BMI	Date	Weight	BMI

4.31 KEEP A MONTHLY MEASUREMENT CHART

Give yourself a gold star when you go down one size!

Date	Chest/Bust	Waist	Hips	Upper Arm	Thigh	Calf

1. Introduction

- It's true; we are what we eat. So, starting now, resolve to be in charge of what you eat. Become one of the healthy attitude people who eat to live, not who live to eat.
- Following a healthy diet helps us to look better, feel better, and stay healthy.
- Realize you might need to change or at least modify your eating habits and style.
- Trust your instincts. You know more than you think you do.
- You already know that you must eat fewer calories and work out more for the pounds to come off.
- You know you must lose weight slowly—on average 1 1/2 to 2 lbs. a week—for the weight to stay off.

2. Commit To A Healthier Lifestyle And Eat A Healthy Diet

- Along with those leftover potato chips, toss that hidden pack of cigarettes, limit alcohol consumption, get plenty of rest, exercise daily and try to minimize stress.
- Don't try to lose weight too quickly.
- The healthiest and longest lasting weight loss occurs slowly.
- If you lose one to two pounds each week, you are more apt to keep the weight off.

3. Information & Knowledge

- Start only when you're ready, when you have a plan, and all the pieces are in place. Don't start when you're depressed on in the middle of a major life change.
- If you're trying a particular diet, make sure to read about it first. It's easy to gain weight on the Zone Diet or the Atkins if you're not doing them correctly.
- *STIKKY Weight Management and the American Diabetes Assn. Complete Weight Loss Workbook* are super informative and very clear. (See Resources in the back of the book.)

4. Determination

- Make the commitment.
- Look in the mirror and call the police—or take the vow and start *now*.
- Build a base of Can-Do's.

5. Fad Diets

- Send you into a cycle of quick weight loss and rebound weight (gain back what you lost plus five pounds) making it harder the next time you try to lose weight.
- People do lose weight on crash diets, but no one seems to lose weight "sensibly," that is, permanently, or healthfully.
- But hey, some people only learn by banging their head against a wall.

6. Starvation Works — But Only Temporarily

- It's not healthy and your body makes every effort to thwart you.
- It slows down your metabolism, causing you to conserve the very fat you are starving yourself to lose.
- And, of course, when you find that you just can't starve yourself anymore, your body will breathe a sigh of relief, put the weight back on and add 5 extra pounds for good measure (called rebound weight), just in case you ever get the silly idea to starve yourself again.

7. Beware of Magic

- Losing weight, exercising regularly, reducing stress are all noble goals but they can be accomplished only if we respect the effort involved.
- Words like *easy, miraculous, breakthrough, remarkable new discovery, 100% guaranteed...* well, if it sounds like snake oil, it is snake oil.

8. Keep it Simple

- Definitely avoid quick-fix schemes, but also stay clear of complex regimens. They're full of pitfalls. One slip and you're a goner.
- Instead, make modest changes to your daily routine; keep them in place until they become a habit—something you do automatically without thinking—then add something else you think will work well.

9. If You've Got It, Use It

- Apply the knowledge you gain.
- A healthy diet and regular exercise are the basics for maintaining a healthy weight, but let's not kid ourselves, losing weight requires additional effort.

10. Hold Steady

- Avoid the roller-coaster ride of your weight going up and down.
- If you simply must, plan one treat or cheat meal a week so you don't go insane from indulgence deprivation.

11. Getting Started — Solicit Help

- A strong support system helps you start off confident you're on the right track.
- Consult with professionals. Up front and personal help from professionals can help you make a strong start.
- A registered dietitian, a fitness expert, and your physician can help you to create and maintain a realistic exercise and nutrition program.
- Make sure you follow your doctor's advice and follow any recommended diet or exercise restrictions.
- Enlist the help of family and friends. If you eat better, so will your family, and your friends might follow your lead as well.

12. Your Ideal Weight

- Remember your ideal weight is primarily your healthiest weight.
- Do not try to become as thin as possible.
- Just like you, yourself, your body is unique. Learn it's strengths and accept any imperfections.
- Other people seldom notice our shortcomings unless we point them out.
- Learn to dress to your strengths, not to the latest fashion trends.
- Be specific in stating your body changing goals (pounds, sizes or both).
- A smaller size of clothing reflects both weight loss and increased muscle from exercise.
- Trying to fit into a favorite dress in time for a big event is a good motivator so long as you don't heave a sigh of relief when it's over and go back to poor eating habits.

13. Goal Setting

- Set realistic and gradual goals.
- Think both short term and long term. 1 1/2 pounds a week = 6 pounds a month = 72 lbs. a year.
- We don't become overweight overnight, so allow sufficient time for healthy weight loss.

14. Make the Best Choice – Make the Healthy Choice

- Doing the best thing is easy. Figuring out what is the best thing to do is hard.
- The closer the food is to the original source the more nutritious and least fattening it will be.
- High fiber food like fruits, vegetables, legumes and whole grains fill you up and satisfy your hunger more than highly processed foods.
- Limit your intake of saturated fat. Choose lean meats and substitute non-saturated fats (oils) for butter.
- Eat at least five servings each of fresh fruits and fresh or lightly cooked vegetables each day.
- Avoid or cut out the white powders—salt, sugar and flour. A friend refers to them as the cocaine of the food industry.
- Experts warn that high-fructose corn syrup is making us fat.
- Try eating smaller meals more often—4-6 times a day. The key word here is *smaller*!

15. Yes, Calories Still Count — So Count 'Em

- Keep your calorie count in line with your weight loss goals.
- Choose "quality" calories over "empty" ones.
- Avoid high calorie foods such as cheese, butter, whole milk, red meat, and sweets.
- Although the formula is simple—energy expenditure must exceed energy intake—putting it into practice is hard work.

16. Reading the Menu as a Process of Elimination

- Prepare in advance for eating away from home. Decide if you want American, Chinese, Mexican, Italian, etc.
- Decide before you open the menu:
    if you're going to have a full meal or something light.
    if you want vegetarian or meat.
    if you want beef, pork, veal, lamb, chicken, duck, etc.
- When you're pretty sure you know what you want, open the menu and pick the better of the first two items.
- Go to the next item and compare it with what you've already preferred.
- Keep going until you finish reading the menu and you'll wind up with your final best choice.
- It might take you a couple of times to perfect this method, but you'll get really fast at making the best choice—something delicious that is also healthful.
- Here's an idea from americaonthemove.org for stopping weight gain—eat 100 fewer calories a day and take 2000 more steps (a mile) than usual.

17. Controlling Portions

- Eat smaller portions. *Everyone who is overweight eats too much* so cut back—way back.
- Cutting down rather than eliminating your favorite foods will be better in the long run.
- Be suspicious of the term "serving size" on food labels. *No one* eats these quantities.
- The information *is* useful, however, to get a fix on how much salt, sugar, calories, fat, etc.

it contains. Multiply it by 3 if *your* usual helping is 3 times what is recommended for a serving.
- Don't guess. Precisely measure and weigh what you actually eat.
- Use the following guidelines from the American Institute for Cancer Research for determining portion sizes.

> Chopped vegetables: 1/2 cup (a rounded handful)
> Raw leafy vegetables: 1 cup (the size of an adult fist)
> Fresh fruit: one medium fruit (or 1/2 cup chopped)
> Dried fruit: 1/4 cup (the size of a golf ball)
> Pasta or rice (cooked): 1/2 cup (rounded handful)
> Nuts: 1/3 cup (a level handful)
> Cheese: 1/1/2 ounces (a cube slightly larger than 1 square inch)
> Meat: the size of a deck of cards
> Cereal: 1/2 cup
> Juice: 6 ounces
> Milk: 8 ounces
> Salt: minimum amounts
> Sugar: minimum amounts

18. Plan Ahead
- Keep healthful foods on hand for snacking.
- Keep healthful food visible—on the table, in the fridge.
- Ahead of time, decide what you will do when a feast appears miraculously in front of you.
- Stock your refrigerator and cupboards with healthful foods. Because unhealthful (high-calorie, fats, sugars, salts) are the quickest and easiest to prepare, it's important to not have them available.

19. Pre-Prepare
- Your number one job every evening will be to plan tomorrow's meals.
- Before you go to bed make sure you know when and what you're going to eat the next day and do any required prep work and lunch packing.
- As we all well know, it's hard to stay motivated when we're tired and sleepy.

20. Food Shopping
- Shop only with a full stomach. If you're hungry you'll buy everything in sight.
- Shop from a list.

21. Food Preparation
- Trim excess fat from meat and remove poultry skin before cooking.

22. Uncle Charlie says:
- "The other half of this sandwich is probably going to taste just like the first half. I think I'll just wrap it up and eat it later when I'm hungry."
- When offered seconds he usually says, "No thanks. I'm just taking in enough fuel to fly me home."

23. Serving Food
- Serve cafeteria style — from the stove. Dishes of food on the table make everyone reach for more.

24. Meals
- Don't skip meals. Be a clock watcher. Eating at set times keeps your appetite and food choices under control.
- Try to consume more of your calories earlier in the day. (Breakfast like a king, lunch like a prince, sup like a pauper.)
- Eating breakfast helps increase your metabolism early in the day; thus you burn more calories.
- Eat fruit instead of fruit juice.
- If it tastes good, spit it out.

25. Fool the Eye
- Use one size smaller bowls and plates—luncheon plate for dinner, dessert bowl for cereal, etc. Your servings will appear larger on smaller dishes.
- Use a salad fork and a teaspoon; they will force you to take smaller bites.

26. Re-learn How to Eat
- Eat slowly. You'll eat less, because your "I'm full" signal will go off sooner.
- Focus on what you're eating. Don't read, watch TV or do the crossword–just eat.
- Put down your fork/spoon between bites.

27. Water
- Drink eight to ten 8-ounce glasses of water each day; it flushes toxins from your system.
- Drink water instead of sodas and fruit juice.
- Two other reasons for drinking lots of water—you'll fool your body into thinking it's full and improve your complexion at the same time.

28. Vitamins
- Take a daily multivitamin.

29. Write it Down
- People who keep track every day have a 90% success rate of weight loss.
- Keep a diet journal. This is a great way to stay focused while keeping track of caloric intake and every other aspect of your diet efforts.
- Record your eating habits and exercise activities.
- 100% Chart – Keep track – daily, weekly, monthly, note cause and effect.
- Examine patterns and behaviors in your eating.
- Keep tabs on all small and large successes. Continue to increase awareness.

30. Exercise
- Exercise on an empty, or almost empty, stomach if you can (diabetics usually can't). You'll burn more calories.

31. Habits
- Use the 21 days trick to cut out sugar. Take it one day at a time but stick with it and after three weeks you will find yourself out of the habit of wanting sweets.
- Build a good habits base.

32. Ride Out Food Cravings
- Distinguish hunger from food cravings.
- Be aware when they hit but hold steady; they usually pass in a minute.

33. Forgive Yourself for Backsliding
- Cope positively with slips and relapses into old patterns.
- Take note of what happened, don't dwell on what went wrong, learn from it and pick your program back up again just where you left off.

34. More Exercise
- Exercise aerobically at lest three times a week for a minimum of 15-20 minutes.
- It seems like a no-brainer, but exercise is often ignored in the weight-loss game. At the very least, a brisk hour-long walk will boost most metabolisms and cause a body to burn calories more aggressively throughout the day.

35. Scale
- Weigh yourself only once a week if you can stand not to peek.
- The results are more dramatic if you can resist the daily weigh-in. And you'll cut down on the minute by minute news and self criticism.
- Weight normally varies from day to day, but in a week the general trend is down if you stay righteous.

36. Keep the Faith
- You can do it. Others have; you can, too. Just remember, nobody's perfect. Pretty good is plenty good enough. Good enough is better than nothing at all. We are women (hear us roar) and we are stout hearted men! We will survive. (If we can just avoid more clichés.)

Getting Started with your Goals for:

Reduced Stress   Ideal Weight   Optimal Energy

Motivation

- If not you, who? If not now, when?
- If not you, who? If not now, when?
- Say Yes to better health, normal weight, looking good.
- Dream big to get smaller.
- Do what's right for *you*; this *is* personal.
- Be the Little Engine That Could. "I think I can, I think I can."

Take The Pledge

- Make the decision to get healthy.
- Decide to change the way you eat.
- Promise yourself and one other person you're going to do this and keep plugging away until you succeed.
- Get ready, get set, go!

Learnings — Get The Facts

- Understanding nutrition (we are what we eat),
- Gather information; keep adding to your data base. This is a big thing you're doing. It's going to take a lot of different skills. Learn from your mistakes, sure, but learn from others as well.
- Add to your skill base daily. Notice and appreciate every small success, every good idea, every clever recipe, every new and more pleasant place to walk, every new blossom on the trees you pass. Smile and greet people. Let them know you know their secret — they're human and appreciate a warm smile or a small kindness.
- Commit basic information to memory – Know that a teaspoon of salt has 590 milograms of sodium, that a tablespoon is about the size of your thumb, a serving of meat is the size of a deck of cards, a soda has 150 calories, etc.

Set Real Goals

- Be practical

Set Priorities And Stick With Them.

- Decide what you must do, when you must do those things, and how to schedule enough time to do them. Then arrange other tasks around those must-dos.

Get Onto A Schedule.

- Doing some things at the same time, whether it's daily, weekly, or monthly, means that they get done. Getting into a routine saves time and stress.

Make A Plan

- Make a plan using your current knowledge – you know more than you think you do.
- Include the answers to the questions *who, what, when, where, how, why*?

Calories In / Calories Used — It's About The Balance
- The core of your plan will be specific activities that will help you attain the appropriate balance of calories consumed and calories used.
- How you do this is up to you—after all, this is your plan.

How Other People Lose Weight
- Many people lose weight with well-known diet systems like Weight Watchers, Adkins, South Beach, The Zone, Overeaters Anonymous, Dr. Phil, etc.
- Caution. Read about these systems first. Become informed. If you just start off half cocked, you could gain weight.
- Half the people who have qualified for the National Weight Off Registry (of successful weight loss of more than 30 lbs. kept off for more than a year) had help losing, and half did it all on their own. (Their average weight loss is 60 lbs. and their average time for keeping it off is 5 years.)

Ask Before You Sign On
Dieting programs can be expensive in terms of time and money so it's important to become informed before selecting a given program. Before you sign up with a specific diet program, or decide to follow a program outlined in a book or on the internet, ask some important questions:
- Are there risks? Does it have your doctor's O.K.?
- What proof is there of your program's success?
- What is the success rate of dieters' keeping off the weight they lose?
- How much does it really cost? Are there weekly or yearly fees, charges for food or supplements? Are any costs covered by health insurance?
- If counseling is offered, is there an extra charge?
- If there is a maintenance program after the weight is lost, what are the costs, if any?
- What are the credentials of those who supervise the program on site, and are they trained in CPR?

Establishing Good Habits, One at a Time
- Habits take 21 days to form.
- Don't always make your bed? Wish you did? Would you prefer to come home to a tidy bed in the evening instead of crawling into a crumpled mess? Try this for 21 days. Make your bed as soon as you get up. You will discover that after 21 days you will find yourself, forever and a day, making your bed—happily and unconsciously. Don't believe us, try it.

Make The Best Choice
- Make it a habit to always make the best choice.
  1. Become conscious of the choices open to you.
  2. Remember your pledge to always make the best choice.
- Sample: You can select:
  1. Regular coke (w/sugar and calories)
  2. Diet coke (w/no sugar and w/chemicals)
  3. Water

One Day At A Time
- Plan every 24 hour period carefully (that's a day, you know).
- List your priorities.
- Concentrate on reducing stress, enjoying physical activity, meal preparation, mental attitude, productivity, social interactions, record keeping and planning, relaxation, rest & sleep.

Keep Track
- Pay Attention—daily, weekly, monthly, yearly.
- Keep track of how well you keep to your plan and how effective it is.
- Notice everything, even your mistakes, but only hold onto your successes. Mull them over and enjoy them as you learn from them and vow to continue on your positive path.

Re-Evaluate Regularly — Make Only Small Changes
- Make changes to your plan *slowly*.
- Only one change at a time.
- Only after you're very positive it will be helpful and won't disrupt what you've already got in place.

Stick To It
- Keep your eye on the prize.
- Reward yourself – daily, weekly, monthly, yearly.
- Stick to your original plan for 3 weeks (3 weeks make a habit).

Get Back On The Wagon
- Pick yourself up, dust yourself off, and start all over again.

Do What Works
- If you're a talker, talk about losing weight—talk, but then do!
- If you're more of a super spy type, plan your strategies in secret.

Reduce Stress By Careful And Consistent Planning
- Shopping
- Food preparation
- Making ahead
- Storage

PART 4.4
SUBSTANCE ABUSE/ADDICTIONS

Note: Be sure to make copies of all blank charts before using.

SUBSTANCE ABUSE / ADDICTIONS

The term *substance abuse* describes the misuse of legal substances such as alcoholic beverages, prescription and over-the-counter drugs, and other substances (such as glue), and the illegal use of substances such as street drugs. Substance abuse isn't only a problem of the young; it can occur at any age.

Addiction
According to the dictionary, an addiction is a physical or psychological dependence on a substance or practice that is beyond voluntary control. This definition covers a wide variety of substances—tobacco, alcohol, and drugs (both prescription and illegal).

What's wrong with sipping a beer, taking a muscle relaxant, having a cigarette break or even sharing a joint or a Snickers bar? They all provide pleasure and help us feel better. The trouble seems to be that these seemingly small indulgences can lead to addiction in some people and their bodies eventually need these casual pleasures in order to function. When this happens we have an addition, a compulsive need for a *habit-forming* substance.

Two Significant Characteristics of Addiction
Withdrawal Symptoms occur when an addicted person stops taking the drug on which the body has become dependent. The body reacts with symptoms such as aches and pains, trembling, vomiting, sweating, insomnia, and diarrhea.

Tolerance means that over time the addicted person needs increasing amounts of a substance to experience the same effects. For example, a person who needs twice as many drinks to feel intoxicated has built up a tolerance to alcohol.

Awareness
It's fairly easy to identify people with a drug or alcohol problem. They usually try to hide the common signs (getting high or drunk on a regular basis) and deny the problem in many ways. They lie to themselves and to others about the amount of drugs or alcohol being used, and they prefer the company of fellow addicts, so they can feel comfortable getting drunk or high.

It's almost impossible to hide a cigarette habit but most heavy smokers pretend to smoke less than a pack a day. (Who knew Jackie Kennedy was such a heavy smoker?) As their addiction worsens smokers tend to smoke more in private and pretend to have a bad cold when their smoker's cough becomes impossible to repress.

In Addition to Secretiveness, Other Indicators Are:
- Talking constantly about drugs and alcohol
- Sunglasses when there's no obvious need
- Associating with known substance abusers
- Mood swings and depression; temper, flare-ups
- Getting into legal trouble
- Borrowing money or stealing
- Neglecting responsibilities
- Deterioration of physical appearance
- Missing work or school because of drinking or drug use
- Sudden changes—at work, at school, lower quality of work, lack of discipline
- Pressing others to join them in *enjoying* drugs, alcohol, and even cigarettes
- Secretive behavior, frequent trips to out of the way areas (basement, storeroom, restroom, etc.)

4.4a CO-DEPENDENCY / ENABLING

The word codependency is used to explain a common relationship between a person who is addicted (to alcohol, drugs, gambling, sex, etc.) and another person who is obsessed with controlling the addictive behavior and/or curing the addict's problems. The term has evolved to describe people who see themselves as rescuers of another person engaged in persistent destructive behavior. Codependents cover up the addictive behavior and make excuses for the person, enabling him or her to continue without suffering the normal consequences of the destructive behavior.

While often seen to be angry, controlling, preachy, blaming, or subtly manipulative, codependents are usually frustrated and miserable. If you answer yes to one or more of the following questions, you might need help in learning to detach yourself from the addicted person's life.

Co-Dependency / Enabling Questionaire

	YES	NO
1. Do you hope that your help will change the behavior of a loved one who is addicted or acts compulsively?	_____	_____
2. Do you do more than your share of the work, allowing that person to get by with doing less than his/her share?	_____	_____
3. Do you consistently give more than you receive in the relationship?	_____	_____
4. Do you try to "fix" others' feelings that make you uncomfortable?	_____	_____
5. Do you make excuses for the other person's behavior?	_____	_____
6. Do you try to protect him/her from the consequences of his/her behavior?	_____	_____

Making it Better
An excellent resource is *Codependent No More: How to Stop Controlling Others and Start Caring for Yourself*, 2nd edition by Melody Beattie. Hazelden Educational Materials, 1996.

Treatment for addiction is accomplished mainly through outside help. It is very difficult to *go cold turkey*. The good news is that because the problem is so widespread there are numerous resources. Counseling can be done privately, in a group or even within the family.

Common sources of help include family doctors, clerics, community drug hotlines, local emergency health clinics, community treatment services, local health departments, Alcoholics Anonymous, Narcotics Anonymous, Al-Anon/Alateen (extremely helpful to families of alcoholics).

For additional information about managing addiction, contact the National Clearinghouse for Alcohol and Drug Information, Drug Abuse Information and Treatment Referral Line, P.O. Box 2345, Rockville, MD 0847-2345; 800-662-4357 or 301-468-6433; or visit them online at **www.health.org**.

SMOKING

Most of us have friends and family members who have stopped smoking. We also know people who were not able to stop, or who stopped and then started again. Smoking is a powerful addiction and the effort to stop is an extraordinary one, an effort that is often made more than once.

The nicotine in cigarettes is highly addictive and can create a dependence that triggers withdrawal symptoms ranging from insomnia and changes in heart rate to chills and fever, anxiety, nausea, and cravings for tobacco (which can last a lifetime for some people).

Smoking kills by contributing to a wide range of health problems, including emphysema, heart disease, and lung cancer.

Although smoking is on the decrease in the US there are still 50 million smokers and it is on the increase in children.
- Smoking causes almost 90% of lung cancer.
- Heavy smoking attacks women's reproductive systems.
- Smoking *seriously* increases problems with blood vessels that are caused by heart disease and diabetes.
- Smoking makes you ugly. It damages the small blood vessels in the skin causing early wrinkles and fine lines, especially around the eyes.
- Severe dental problems are four times more likely in smokers.

Knowing All This, Why Don't We Quit?
We try. But cigarettes are so excruciatingly addictive that smokers tend to attempt to quit once, twice, and many times over, with varying degrees of success. Statistics differ. One source says only one in 40 smokers is successful at quitting. Another says seven out of a hundred make it. These are appalling odds. It's obvious that trying to quit is much harder than is commonly thought. Going cold turkey is the most common effort and has the highest failure rate.

Why Is It So Hard to Quit?
The chemistry of the brain is altered by long term smoking and willpower alone cannot overcome the hold nicotine has over the smoker. Who has the toughest job to quit? Smokers who have a cigarette the minute their eyes open in the morning, who smoke more than a pack a day, and/or who have tried to quit before and failed. They can all increase their chance of success significantly by weaning themselves off nicotine slowly. More help is needed, however, for a completely realized stop. A counselor can help create a plan, and show how to gain awareness of why you smoke by keeping track of such details as where and when you smoke, and what your feelings are before and after a cigarette.

What Happens When We Quit—The Really Good News Is
We get thanks from the heart immediately, and also from the lungs—eventually. Carbon monoxide levels in the body drop substantially the very day you quit smoking. Within seven days your risk of dying from a sudden heart attack begins a decline that will eventually put you in the same reduced risk level as people who have never smoked. It takes years for the lungs to recover from heavy smoking, but they do recover. They eventually get back that healthy pink color.

You'll get a jump start if you *hit the ground running*. Really. If you begin a regular exercise program you are 50% more likely to kick the smoking habit permanently.

RESOURCES TO STOP SMOKING

The American Cancer Society (800-227-2345) and the American Lung Association (800-586-5872) are excellent sources of support and information for those looking to quit on their own. Also, smoking treatment programs in your area are listed in the Yellow Pages.

Other sources of help are books, the Internet and your doctor. We recommend you research carefully, make a strong plan, try to take a deep breath and get ready for success.

Your Doctor Can Be a Big Help
A number of smoking cessation products are now available to help break the smoking habit— nicotine patches, nicotine gum, and drugs such as Zyban, an antidepressant that has recently been approved for use in smoking cessation. These products provide a low dose of nicotine that can be used to wean the body away from the drug. Most require a physician's prescription.

Books
7 Steps to a Smoke-Free Life. John Wiley & Sons, 1998. Uses the *Freedom from Smoking* program of the American Lung Association.

Web Sites
www.lungusa.org is the web site of the American Lung Association, 1740 Broadway, NY, NY 10019, 202/315-8700. Find the *Freedom from Smoking* program on their web site for a seven-part program that will motivate you and show you how to quit. It is considered the best smoking-cessation program available.

www.nicotine-anonymous.org offers a 12-step program to help smokers quit.

www.quitsmoking.com provides products for sale (hence the **.com** of their web site address) but they also provide helpful information.

www.commitlozenge.com offers information about the Commit lozenge.

www.quit.com also has information about stopping smoking.

Additional resources for stopping smoking can be found in the back of the book.

When monitoring your progress think in terms of baby steps. The reason we smile and applaud the baby's first steps is that it is a big deal to begin to walk. And it is a big deal for you when you begin to quit! Don't ignore the failures but focus on the successes. Note your efforts, problems, successes, feelings, new ideas, new learnings, etc.

6 a.m. _____

7 a.m. _____

8 a.m. _____

9 a.m. _____

10 a.m. _____

11 a.m. _____

12 a.m. _____

1 p.m. _____

2 p.m. _____

3 p.m. _____

4 p.m. _____

5 p.m. _____

6 p.m. _____

7 p.m. _____

8 p.m. _____

9 p.m. _____

10 p.m. _____

11 p.m. _____

12 p.m. _____

1 a.m. _____

2 a.m. _____

3 a.m. _____

4 a.m. _____

5 a.m. _____

Remember a log is sequential and ongoing. It answers the fact
questions—*who, what, when, where, how* and *why*.

4.4c SMOKING JOURNAL

Write down anything relevant to your smoking habit, insights, triggers, costs, work or home problems. Stick to the fact questions and you will be amazed at the insight you will gain when you go back a day later and read your notes.

_____
_____
_____
_____
_____
_____
_____
_____
_____
_____
_____
_____
_____
_____
_____
_____
_____
_____
_____
_____
_____
_____
_____
_____
_____
_____
_____
_____
_____
_____
_____
_____
_____
_____
_____
_____
_____
_____
_____
_____

4.4d   SMOKING CESSATION EFFORTS

In this log keep track of:
- Doctor's Office Visits/Procedures
- Medications/Over the Counter Drugs
- X Rays
- Group Efforts
- Surgeries
- Allergic Reactions
- Cancer Alerts
- Successes

Date	Event	Physician/Facility
Rx	Treatment	Results

_____
_____
_____
_____
_____
_____
_____
_____
_____
_____
_____
_____
_____
_____
_____
_____
_____
_____
_____
_____
_____
_____
_____
_____
_____
_____
_____
_____
_____

Remember a log is sequential and ongoing. It answers the fact
questions—*who, what, when, where, how* and *why*.

4.4 e ALCOHOL ABUSE QUIZ

Most of us have friends and family members who have stopped drinking. We also know people who were not able to stop, or who stopped and then started again. Alcohol is a powerful addiction and the effort to overcome it is an extraordinary one, an effort that is often made more than once.

Initial efforts to overcome alcohol abuse are like baby steps—awkward and halting at first and all of a sudden we're flying along and everyone who loves us shouts, "Hurrah!" at our success. During the process, while it's important to notice when we fail, the real focus is on every success, large or small.

Giving up alcohol entails setting long term goals but filling in with reachable interim goals and paying close attention to each hour of each day as we get free of the curse alcohol has placed on our lives.

It's not as easy to identify alcoholism as it is, say, smoking addiction. Most people who drink (one or two drinks enjoyed now and then) are considered moderate drinkers. *Alcohol abuse* is characterized by drinking in large amounts or in binges. And there are serious personal and social consequences that result.

Quiz

Answering the following questions might help you to identify whether you have a drinking problem. There's room to elaborate on your answers.

1. Have you ever felt you ought to cut down on your drinking?_____
_____

2. Have people annoyed you by criticizing your drinking?_____
_____

3. Have you ever felt bad or guilty about your drinking? _____
_____

4. Have you ever had a drink first thing in the morning (an eye opener) to steady your nerves or get rid of a hangover?_____
_____

If you answered *yes* to one or more of the first three questions, you may be developing a drinking problem. A yes answer to the fourth question is a sign of a more serious problem that should be treated.

Additional Signs of a Drinking Problem Include:

• Missing work or being late to work because of a hangover_____
_____

• Not being able to perform housework or daily tasks _____
_____

• Having memory lapses or blackouts _____
_____

• Having sexual relations with someone to whom you wouldn't ordinarily be attracted
_____

- Fighting with your spouse or friends or hitting your children _____
  _____

- Being preoccupied with drinking and organizing activities and social functions
  around alcohol _____

- Having marriage or family problems in which drinking could be a factor _____
  _____

- Having an auto accident after leaving a party in an intoxicated state _____
  _____

Your honest answers to these tough questions should help you decide whether or not you
need help. Some people benefit from joining Alcoholics Anonymous, Al-anon, Al-teen, or the
National Association of Children of Alcoholics, psychiatrists, psychologists, and social workers
provide professional treatment for alcohol abuse.

*Note: Spouses who have been asked to fill out the questionnaire as well, have been
known to shed a bright light.*

BEST RESOURCES TO STOP DRINKING

Alcoholics Anonymous (AA) has the most success with abetting alcohol abuse. The most
important aspect of their program seems to be the regular meetings for people who have made
the decision to attempt to stop drinking and who are looking for help to do it. AA also has very
successful programs for family members who want to gain information on how to do an
intervention, an attempt by family and friends of alcoholics to bring the alcoholic to a decision
to try to stop.

*Note: "Is your life affected by someone's drinking? To help them, you have to help
yourself first." Call Al-Anon/Alateen, 888-425-2666 or www.al-anon.alateen.org.*

Use this log to gain self-knowledge. When monitoring your progress think in terms of baby steps. The reason we smile and applaud the baby's first steps is that it is a big deal to begin to walk. And it is a big deal for you when you begin to quit! Don't ignore the failures but focus on the successes. Note your efforts, problems, successes, feelings, new ideas, new learnings, etc.

6 a.m.   _____

7 a.m.   _____

8 a.m.   _____

9 a.m.   _____

10 a.m.   _____

11 a.m.   _____

12 a.m.   _____

1 p.m.   _____

2 p.m.   _____

3 p.m.   _____

4 p.m.   _____

5 p.m.   _____

6 p.m.   _____

7 p.m.   _____

8 p.m.   _____

9 p.m.   _____

10 p.m.   _____

11 p.m.   _____

12 p.m.   _____

1 a.m.   _____

2 a.m.   _____

3 a.m.   _____

4 a.m.   _____

5 a.m.   _____

Remember a log is sequential and ongoing.
It answers the fact questions: *who, what, when, where, how and why.*

4.4 g DRINKING JOURNAL

Write down anything relevant to your drinking habit—insights, triggers, costs, work or home problems. Stick to the fact questions and you will be amazed at the insight you will gain when you go back a day later and read your notes.

_____
_____
_____
_____
_____
_____
_____
_____
_____
_____
_____
_____
_____
_____
_____
_____
_____
_____
_____
_____
_____
_____
_____
_____
_____
_____
_____
_____
_____
_____
_____
_____
_____
_____
_____
_____
_____
_____
_____
_____

4.4 h   KEEP TRACK OF YOUR EFFORTS TO STOP DRINKING

- Doctor's Office Visits/Procedures
- Medications/Over the Counter Drugs
- X Rays
- Group Efforts

- Surgeries
- Allergic Reactions
- Cancer Alerts
- Successes

Date   Event   Physician/Facility
Rx   Treatment   Results

_____
_____
_____
_____
_____
_____
_____
_____
_____
_____
_____
_____
_____
_____
_____
_____
_____
_____
_____
_____
_____
_____
_____
_____
_____
_____
_____
_____
_____
_____

Remember a log is sequential and ongoing. It answers the fact
questions—*who, what, when, where, how* and *why*.

ABUSE OF PRESCRIPTION & ILLEGAL DRUGS

Some of us have friends or family members who have overcome their drug addiction.
We also know people who were not able to stop, or who stopped and then started again. Drugs have a powerful effect on the body, and the effort to overcome this insidious addiction is an extraordinary one, an effort that is usually made more than once.

Possibly more than with any other addiction, intensive, professional, and prolonged help is needed to become drug free and stay drug free.

PRESCRIPTION DRUGS

Many, many people take prescription drugs for non-medical reasons. The most usual ones are drugs that alter mental states, such as tranquilizers, sleeping pills, stimulants, and pain killers. We are all familiar with and appreciative of these drugs and the power they have to help us when we really need them.

Drug Abuse Comes About When We:
>   Increase the dosage of these drugs.
>   Use them for longer than was prescribed.
>   Use them to get high or intoxicated, instead of for medical reasons.

Tranquilizers are used to treat stress or anxiety. Low doses, taken as prescribed, make you feel cheerful and relaxed; high doses can make you feel intoxicated. With repeated use people become *dependent* and if they stop using the drug they most likely experience severe anxiety, nervousness, insomnia or more serious symptoms.

Sleeping Pills (barbiturates and other sedatives) are meant to be used short-term to treat long-term sleeplessness or insomnia. Long-term use may lead to dependency, a need to take ever larger doses to obtain the same effect. Continuous and increasingly stronger use of sleeping pills results in next day *hangover*, dullness, lack of concentration, poor memory, mood swings, depression, irritability and anxiety. Withdrawal symptoms are even more than those associated with stopping tranquilizers.

Amphetamines such as the stimulants Benzedrine and Dexedrine increase energy and decrease appetite. Used in the past for diet pills, they caused people to get *hooked* and to become psychologically and physically dependent. Now they are more often used illegally to enhance the effects of other drugs.

Painkillers prescribed by a physician are typically used to reduce your sensitivity to pain but they also relax you and impart a sense of well-being. They are highly addictive with serious withdrawal symptoms when you try to stop taking them.

NON-PRESCRIPTION DRUGS

Illegal Drugs are used by people of all socioeconomic status, and of all ages, race, and sex, and from all countries. Drug users:

- have a higher incidence of sexually transmitted diseases.
- have poor nutrition, making them at higher risk of other diseases.
- who share needles are at increased risk of getting infections such as HIV (the cause of AIDS) and hepatitis B. Illegal drugs taken during pregnancy may lead to premature birth or death of the fetus. If the baby is born, it may already be addicted.

Narcotics dull the senses, relieve pain, and produce sleep. The most familiar of the illegal narcotics is heroin. Addiction to heroin develops quickly, and chronic use causes serious health problems. Withdrawal symptoms include anxiety, sweating, shaking, cramps, and an intense craving for heroin. Some individuals addicted to heroin are given a synthetic substitute for heroin, methadone, to help them function without the drug.

Cocaine gives an immediate, short-term but intense feeling of well-being, an increase in self-confidence, energy, and sensuality, and decrease in appetite. Because this *high* is followed by a low, the user soon wants to take more, leading to addiction. The most popular form of cocaine—*crack*—is the most addictive. The physical effects of cocaine put a strain on the body that can lead to chest pain, heart attack, stroke, seizures, or convulsions.

Hallucinogens such as marijuana, LSD, and PCP (angel dust), affect the central nervous system, change a person's ability to understand, and alter body function. In addition to producing a relaxed and detached mood and an altered sense of time, marijuana also can impair memory, the ability to think logically, and coordination. Chronic heavy use results in a loss of energy and drive and may lead to psychological dependence. PCP and LSD, on the other hand, usually produce more vivid, unpredictable responses, which can lead to flashbacks, violence, and chronic mental disorders.

Resources for substance abuse can be found in the back of the book.

When monitoring your progress think in terms of baby steps. The reason we smile and applaud the baby's first steps is that it is a big deal to begin to walk. And it is a big deal for you when you begin to quit! Don't ignore the failures but focus on the successes. Note your efforts, problems, successes, feelings, new ideas, new learnings, etc.

6 a.m. _____

7 a.m. _____

8 a.m. _____

9 a.m. _____

10 a.m. _____

11 a.m. _____

12 a.m. _____

1 p.m. _____

2 p.m. _____

3 p.m. _____

4 p.m. _____

5 p.m. _____

6 p.m. _____

7 p.m. _____

8 p.m. _____

9 p.m. _____

10 p.m. _____

11 p.m. _____

12 p.m. _____

1 a.m. _____

2 a.m. _____

3 a.m. _____

4 a.m. _____

5 a.m. _____

4.4 j   DRUG USE JOURNAL

Write down anything relevant to your drug use habit, insights, triggers, costs, work or home problems. Stick to the fact questions and you will be amazed at the insight you will gain when you go back a day later and read your notes.

_____
_____
_____
_____
_____
_____
_____
_____
_____
_____
_____
_____
_____
_____
_____
_____
_____
_____
_____
_____
_____
_____
_____
_____
_____
_____
_____
_____
_____
_____
_____
_____
_____
_____
_____
_____
_____
_____
_____

4.4k   DRUG USE CESSATION EFFORTS

In this log keep track of:
- Doctor's Office Visits/Procedures
- Medications/Over the Counter Drugs
- X Rays
- Group Efforts
- Surgeries
- Allergic Reactions
- Cancer Alerts
- Successes

Date	Event	Physician/Facility
Rx	Treatment	Results

_____

_____

_____

_____

_____

_____

_____

_____

_____

_____

_____

_____

_____

_____

_____

_____

_____

_____

_____

_____

_____

_____

_____

_____

_____

_____

_____

_____

_____

_____

Remember a log is sequential and ongoing. It answers the fact
questions—*who, what, when, where, how* and *why*.

PART 5
HOSPITALS

Note: Be sure to make copies of all blank charts before using.

HOSPITALS

If you need hospital care, you will most likely be ill and not fully able to care for yourself. We'll fervently hope you find yourself in an excellent hospital, of which there are many. Here's what you can do to help manage the episode.

Make Detailed Notes Every Time You Go to the Hospital
- If you think it's necessary, have a trusted family member or close friend help you with this.
- If you can't take your Red Notebook with you, buy a red spiral school notebook and *tape Hospital Log Chart 5a* or *Surgery Log 5c* on the inside front cover.

Write down all the *facts* surrounding each medical event:
- Hospitalization
- Surgery
- Medical Procedure
- Emergency
- Out-Patient Treatment

Record specifics:
- Date
- Treatment
- Results
- Medications
- Hospital name
- Test
- Follow-up
- Area or department of the hospital where you are treated
- Reason for being at the hospital
- Procedure
- Key personnel

• Try to write down **the name of every doctor** who sees you (ask for their cards). Usually, in a hospital setting, more than one doctor will be involved so it's important to keep track of who sees you and why. Usually the attending physician is the doctor who has the main responsibility for your care whereas "consultants" advise in specific areas of expertise. Doctors/residents/medical students may also be involved. More and more a Hospitalist takes on the role of your primary attending physician while you are in the hospital.

• Try to **ask for the name each time a medicine** is given to you. The nurse will be happy to tell you so you can record it. Be accurate about the spelling, the dosage and the time.

• Ask for and **keep copies of all records**, especially bills. You can double-check them against your own log entries. You will be given discharge instructions; review them with the nurse. The doctor will dictate a discharge summary after you have left, but you are entitled to a copy so ask for it. It is particularly important to **keep test results** as a backup for your primary physician. Be sure to ask for them.

Following is a summary of rights which are spelled out in the American Hospital Association's *Patient's Bill of Rights.* You have the right:
- To be spoken to in words you understand and to ask for a clear re-explanation.
- To know exactly what's wrong with you.
- To read your own medical record and/or to have a copy if you wish.
- To know the benefits and risks of any treatment, or alternative treatment.
- To know the costs involved in treatment or tests.
- To participate fully in all medical decisions including the right to refuse any medical procedure offered.

Always ask questions about all instructions, shots and treatments. In the process of answering your questions, hospital staff will automatically double check their procedures and give careful thought to your care and treatment.

For each entry be sure to include: date, event, facility or hospital,
ward, key personnel, treatment, results, comments, etc.

_____
_____
_____
_____
_____
_____
_____
_____
_____
_____
_____
_____
_____
_____
_____
_____
_____
_____
_____
_____
_____
_____
_____
_____
_____
_____
_____
_____
_____
_____
_____

Remember a log is sequential and ongoing. It answers the fact
questions—*who, what, when, where, how* and *why.*

Most hospitals provide a broad range of services which include emergency treatment, out patient procedures, maternity services, intensive care for serious or terminal illness, exploratory or elective surgery, as well as many other services.

At some point most of us have been or will be admitted to the hospital. Stays in the hospital are significantly shorter than in the past. As a matter of fact, patients can expect to be discharged sooner rather than later.

Traditionally the hospital supplies all your needs, including a gown and toiletry articles. However, if there is time to plan for a stay at the hospital, especially if it is to be of some duration, it is more pleasant and convenient to bring certain items from home. Following is a list of items you might want to have with you:

_____	Red spiral notebook	_____	Medicines/prescriptions
_____	Pencil		(inform your hospital physician)
_____	Snacks	_____	Health insurance card
_____	Glasses or Contact lenses	_____	Vitamins/supplements
_____	Laptop & work (if you must)		(inform your hospital physician)
_____	Lens care equipment	_____	Address/phone numbers
_____	Shampoo, rinse	_____	Comb, brush
_____	Mousse, hair spray	_____	Hairdryer
_____	Makeup	_____	Favorite toiletries
_____	Toothbrush, toothpaste	_____	Floss
_____	Lip Balm	_____	Towel, wash cloth, small bar soap
_____	Deodorant	_____	Razor, shaving cream, after shave
_____	Stuffed animal or favorite pillow	_____	Gown, pajamas
_____	Bed jacket or sweater	_____	Bathrobe
_____	Underwear	_____	Socks
_____	Easy-on shoes	_____	Slippers
_____	Thongs for the shower	_____	Clothes to wear home
_____	Books, magazines	_____	Crossword puzzles
_____	Knitting, embroidery, etc.	_____	Handicrafts
_____	C D s	_____	Walkman & tapes
_____	Earplugs		

Be friendly and polite to all hospital staff, especially nurses and aides, who will be the ones actually taking care of you. Their responsibilities include implementing the doctor's orders as well as using their own judgment and up-close knowledge to help doctors decide when to modify treatment. Nurses are usually the ones who go to bat for patients needing special attention, extra pain medicine, etc. They are the ones who assess your day to day health, give medications, help you ambulate post-surgery, adjust your oxygen levels and clean your wounds. Aides are the ones who will help you eat, give you water, and keep you clean and comfortable. It obviously makes sense to be especially appreciative and respectful to your nurses and aides.

Use two or more lines if need be to describe your hospital stay. Be sure to include detailed information including:

- Date
- Emergency or elective
- Primary physician

- Age at time of surgery
- Hospital
- Results

- Name of surgery
- Surgeon
- Complications if any

_____
_____
_____
_____
_____
_____
_____
_____
_____
_____
_____
_____
_____
_____
_____
_____
_____
_____
_____
_____
_____
_____
_____
_____
_____
_____
_____
_____
_____
_____

Remember a log is sequential and ongoing. It answers the fact
questions—*who, what, when, where, how* and *why*.

PART 6
INSURANCE

Note: Be sure to make copies of all blank charts before using.

Before You Need Health Insurance Coverage, Read the Small Print

It is our suspicion that health insurance policies are written specifically so that you cannot understand what kind of coverage you actually have. We further suspect that it is written precisely so you will *not* have the coverage you need when you most need it. Having been totally honest with you, and having removed all hope, we will now try to help you through the maze.

Health insurance is not a thing to be abused, of course, but it does exist to be used when needed. Our basic advice to you is be prepared to fight for your right to have health coverage—when you need it—because you have already paid for it during all the years you did not need it.

Most companies you work for offer health insurance as a benefit. Understand this benefit is *not* a gift but part of your compensation for working for the company. This is an important concept so make sure you are clear about it.

- Ask for detailed brochures, booklets, videos, or any other explanatory materials from your insurer. Preview them at your leisure so that you will be well prepared. Comprehend what you can on your own, then make a list of questions needing clarification.

- Find a person you trust who is able to read your policy or policies and translate them into clear English. You need to understand what your health insurance does, and what it will cover. Ask your translator/instructor to be patient and don't let yourself be rushed.

- If you need further clarification, call your insurance agent or company representative and ask for a sit-down meeting so that all your remaining questions can be answered. Be sure to satisfy yourself that you have a clear overview of your coverage.

- The first step in learning is simply to be able to follow what is being said. The final step—much more difficult—is to turn around and explain it clearly to someone else. You don't really know until you can tell someone else. Take all the time you need to get to this second stage of being informed.

- Make sure you understand what the company will and will not pay for. Know if there are any cash outlay *limits* for items they cover.

- Invest the time beforehand so that you can understand clearly. You don't want to try to figure it out in the middle of an emergency. And remember, it saves you money when you know what you are entitled to have.

BASIC TERMINOLOGY OF HEALTH INSURANCE

Insurance / Annual Deductible
Most policies require an annual deductible (for example $500) before the insurer will begin to reimburse medical expenditures. Caution: make sure your policy doesn't state a deductible for each doctor or medical service, or for each family member. Yes, it happens.

Maximum Lifetime Benefit/Cap
Be sure to find out if there is a *maximum* amount your insurance will pay and what it is.

Co-Insurance (co-payment) & Usual and Customary
Even after the annual deductible has been met, most insurance companies will pay only a percentage of medical costs — usually 80%. If your doctor charges more than the "usual and customary" rate, you will not only pay the 20% co-payment, you'll also be billed for the difference between what your doctor charges and what is considered the "usual and customary" rate. This is a small-print nightmare so try your best to read your insurance policy carefully. Ask your doctor what his rates are in relation to what are called "usual and customary" rates.

Inpatient Benefits / Outpatient Benefits
There is usually a stated flat fee co-pay and co-insurance percentage for inpatient and for outpatient benefits as described above. However, they may not be the same amounts so be sure to check. If it's not clear, ask again.

Prescription Drugs
The flat fee co-pay and co-insurance percentage for prescription drugs might be different from outpatient or inpatient benefits so be sure to check.

MEDICARE/MEDICAID INFORMATION

Online
Information about Social Security insurance can be accessed online at **www.socialsecurity.gov**.

In Person
It's necessary to get in line an hour early and wait for the door to open at 8:00 if you want to speak with a Social Security representative directly and not wait all morning to do so. But it's well worth the effort. They are extremely well informed and helpful and will take the time to make your benefits clear to you.

By Phone
If you call the office, prepare your questions ahead of time and take careful notes. Be sure to note the name of the person you speak with and ask how you might reach the same person the next time you call. Lots of luck.

HEALTH INSURANCE INFORMATION

If you are part of a group plan, ask others in the group what experience they've had with your insurance—surprises, pitfalls, gross injustices, etc.

Why Claims are Denied

1. **Error**—Doctors write in the wrong code for the diagnosis or make some other simple error. This is fairly common so ask for a clear explanation of what happened.

2. **Out of network**—If you select a doctor who is not on your insurer's list, they will likely deny the claim.

3. **Pre-existing conditions**—Read your policy carefully. Some policies define pre-existing when there was no previous diagnosis but only symptoms.

4. **Not medically necessary**—An insurance claims processor can decide the service was not necessary or did not meet some other technicality requirement. Your doctor knows the insurance point of view and if she prescribes the treatment anyway, you should continue to press your claim through an appeals process.

5. **Non-covered benefit**—This is where reading the policy is so difficult. It generally tells you what it covers but not so much what it doesn't. Although your insurance policy includes a list of *not covered*, somehow you don't notice until you require the service and it's not available. You might want to ask up front. "Tell me the most common conditions your policy does not cover and why," is a fair request. Most plans have an appeals process that both you and your doctor can use if you disagree with the plan's findings. Hold off on paying medical bills until you feel the insurance company has paid everything it should.

6. **Seek help**—If your company's provider doesn't meet your family's needs, try to get someone from personnel to champion your cause.

7. **Be persistent**—Don't give up.

The Following Basic Information Should Be Kept With Your Emergency Numbers.

Name of Claimant _____   Effective Date of Insurance _____

Insurance Co. _____
           name   **address**   **contact**   **phone**

Agent's name _____   Phone # _____   Fax # _____

Type of policy (HMO, PPO, Medicare, Medicaid) _____

Group_____   or individual policy? _____   Payor #_____

Employer providing insurance_____   Group # _____

Covered employee_____

Covered employee ID# _____   Relationship to claimant _____

Total monthly premium $ _____   Yearly deductible $ _____

% Deductible per claim_____   Flat fee co-pay per claim $ _____

Claim # _____

If you are part of a group plan, ask others in the group what experience they've had with your insurance—surprises, pitfalls, gross injustices, etc.

The Following Basic Information Should Be Kept With Your Emergency Numbers.

Name of Claimant _____   Effective Date of Insurance _____

Insurance Co. _____
           name   **address**   **contact**   **phone**

Agent's name _____   Phone # _____   Fax # _____

Type of policy (HMO, PPO, Medicare, Medicaid) _____

Group_____   or individual policy?_____   Payor #_____

Employer providing insurance_____   Group # _____

Covered employee_____

Covered employee ID# _____   Relationship to claimant _____

Total monthly premium $ _____   Yearly deductible $ _____

% Deductible per claim_____   Flat fee co-pay per claim $ _____

Claim # _____

If you are part of a group plan, ask others in the group what experience they've had with your insurance—surprises, pitfalls, gross injustices, etc.

Notes:

Outpatient Benefits

Flat Fee—Co-Pay	Co-Insurance % (usually 20%)	
$ _____	$ _____	office visit—primary care physician.
$ _____	$ _____	office visit—specialist physician.
$ _____	$ _____	office visit—outpatient rehabilitation.
$ _____	$ _____	hospital outpatient visit.
$ _____	$ _____	diagnostic testing.
$ _____	$ _____	office visit—outpatient emergency services.
$ _____	$ _____	office visit—mental health visits.
$ _____	$ _____	ambulance service.
$ _____	$ _____	office visit for outpatient surgery.
$ _____	$ _____	wellness care (annual physical, eye exam, etc.)
$ _____	$ _____	dental care.

What Is the Maximum Lifetime Benefit/Cap (if any)? $ _____

Inpatient Benefits

Flat Fee—Co-Pay	Co-Insurance %	
$ _____	$ _____	acute care/inpatient hospital care.
$ _____	$ _____	hospice care.
$ _____	$ _____	a skilled nursing facility..

Prescription Drugs

Flat Fee—Co-Pay	Co-Insurance %	
$ _____	$ _____	brand-name prescription drugs.
$ _____	$ _____	generic prescription drugs.

Additional Questions
- Additional cost to use a doctor outside my plan's network? _____
- Are second opinions covered? _____
- Which hospitals in my area are covered by my plan? _____
- Will home health care be provided if needed? _____
- If so, what is the flat fee co-pay $ _____
  or % co-insurance $ _____
- If I decide on a clinical trial, what, if anything, will my insurance plan cover? _____

Filing Claims
- How do I file claims? _____
- How soon can I expect payment? _____

6c MEDICAL SERVICES NORMALLY COVERED BY HEALTH INSURANCE

Compare this list to what is stated in your policy. Ask questions if you're not sure what is covered.

_____ Doctor's Office visits
_____ Preventive Care
_____ Check Ups
_____ Dental care
_____ Eyeglasses
_____ Contact lenses
_____ Hearing aids
_____ Prosthesis
_____ Artificial limbs
_____ Hospitalizations
_____ Skilled nursing care
_____ Outpatient procedures
_____ Inpatient surgery
_____ Physician hospital visit
_____ Prescription drugs
_____ Lab work
_____ Tests
_____ Procedures
_____ Maternity care
_____ Physical therapy
_____ Speech therapy
_____ Mental health care
_____ Drug and alcohol abuse treatment
_____ Rehabilitation care
_____ Acupuncture
_____ Chiropractic services
_____ Ambulance
_____ Lodging, transportation, & meals while out of town for medical care
_____ Nursing home care
_____ Special care equipment
_____ Home improvements for the disabled
_____ Home health care
_____ Oxygen
_____ Hospice care

Notes:

INSURANCE COMPANY CONTACT

Keep A Written Record Of All Contact With Your Insurance Company.
It will be especially important if there is a discrepancy of any kind.
- All correspondence
- Claims forms
- Copies of bills
- Phone conversations—date and time
  Get the names of the people you speak with, and make a note of the reason for each call—specifically what you talked about, any decisions that were made and any follow-up needed.
- Follow up on agreements
  Double check that referrals have been made, prescriptions have been written, tests and treatments have been scheduled, and all requirements for reimbursements have been met.

Contact the Member Services Division of Your Plan for Information or for a Grievance.
If you have a dispute, you may decide to bring the matter to the attention of:
- Your employee benefits manager.
- Your state insurance commissioner.
- Your state department of health.
- The legal system.

Note: If you are a Medicare or Medicaid beneficiary, there are additional ways to file a grievance. For information, contact your state's Medical Peer Review Organization or State Medicaid Program.

6d   INSURANCE COMPANY CONTACT LOG

Date:_____   Time: _____

Name of phone contact: _____

Question, issue, dispute, or problem being discussed:_____

_____

Outcome:_____

_____

_____

_____

Date:_____   Time: _____

Name of phone contact: _____

Question, issue, dispute, or problem being discussed:_____

_____

Outcome:_____

_____

_____

_____

Date:_____   Time: _____

Name of phone contact: _____

Question, issue, dispute, or problem being discussed:_____

_____

Outcome:_____

_____

_____

_____

Date:_____   Time: _____

Name of phone contact: _____

Question, issue, dispute, or problem being discussed:_____

_____

Outcome:_____

_____

_____

_____

Date:_____   Time: _____

Name of phone contact: _____

Question, issue, dispute, or problem being discussed:_____

_____

Outcome:_____

_____

_____

_____

PART 7
FINANCES

Note: Be sure to make copies of all blank charts before using.

Invoices & Receipts — All Other Financial Papers

Because of the extremely high cost of medical care it is very important to keep close track of your medical expenses and save money wherever possible. Pay only what is owed and make sure you're not billed twice.

Clear and Accurate Record Keeping Is Essential for:

- Filing income taxes
- Receiving insurance reimbursement
- Computing the annual cap on your insurance
- Computing deductible & co-payment costs

Keep all receipts and invoices. If you don't have all the receipts you think you should have, or if you just want to double check your accuracy, call and ask for a duplicate copy of your account sheet from your doctor and/or pharmacist. After entering information on the appropriate *financial chart*, staple all relevant papers together and store them in the *Financial Holding Pouch* at the end of your *Red Notebook*.

State and Federal Income Tax

For tax purposes enter everything in the log and stash all receipts in the Finances Holding Pouch in your Red Notebook. Document all the following expenses:

- Eye glasses
- Prescription drugs
- Medical supplies and equipment
- Transportation to medical services
- Mental illness costs
- Dental expenses
- Your deductible and/or co-pay

> *Note: You can only deduct the amount of medical and dental expenses that exceed 7.5 % of your adjusted gross income. For example, if your adjusted gross income comes to $60,000, you can deduct only those medical expenses over $4,500, which is 7.5% of $60,000.*

Insurance, Annual Deductible

Most policies require an annual deductible (for example $500) before the insurer will begin to reimburse the cost of medical expenditures. Caution: make sure your policy doesn't state a deductible for each separate doctor or medical service, or for each family member. Yes, it happens!

Co-Payment

Even after the annual deductible has been met, most insurance companies will pay only a percentage of medical costs—usually 80%. If your doctor charges more than the "usual and customary" rate, you will not only pay the 20% co-payment, you'll also be billed for the difference between what your doctor charges and what is considered the "usual and customary" rate. This is a small-print nightmare so try your best to read your insurance policy carefully. *Ask your doctor* what his costs are in relation to what are called "usual and customary" rates.

> *Note: Although you cannot deduct the cost of any medical expenses paid by your insurance company or by any other source, or any reimbursements made to you by the insurance company, you should keep an accurate list of them for your own information.*

7a   MEDICAL INSURANCE PREMIUM PAYMENTS
(Only what you pay, not what your employer pays)

Date _____   Paid to _____   Amount paid_____
Date _____   Paid to _____   Amount paid_____
Date _____   Paid to _____   Amount paid_____
Date _____   Paid to _____   Amount paid_____
Date _____   Paid to _____   Amount paid_____
Date _____   Paid to _____   Amount paid_____
Date _____   Paid to _____   Amount paid_____
Date _____   Paid to _____   Amount paid_____
Date _____   Paid to _____   Amount paid_____
Date _____   Paid to _____   Amount paid_____
Date _____   Paid to _____   Amount paid_____
Date _____   Paid to _____   Amount paid_____
Date _____   Paid to _____   Amount paid_____
Date _____   Paid to _____   Amount paid_____
Date _____   Paid to _____   Amount paid_____
Date _____   Paid to _____   Amount paid_____
Date _____   Paid to _____   Amount paid_____
Date _____   Paid to _____   Amount paid_____
Date _____   Paid to _____   Amount paid_____
Date _____   Paid to _____   Amount paid_____
Date _____   Paid to _____   Amount paid_____
Date _____   Paid to _____   Amount paid_____
Date _____   Paid to _____   Amount paid_____
Date _____   Paid to _____   Amount paid_____
Date _____   Paid to _____   Amount paid_____
Date _____   Paid to _____   Amount paid_____
Date _____   Paid to _____   Amount paid_____
Date _____   Paid to _____   Amount paid_____
Date _____   Paid to _____   Amount paid_____
Date _____   Paid to _____   Amount paid_____
Date _____   Paid to _____   Amount paid_____
Date _____   Paid to _____   Amount paid_____
Date _____   Paid to _____   Amount paid_____
Date _____   Paid to _____   Amount paid_____
Date _____   Paid to _____   Amount paid_____
Date _____   Paid to _____   Amount paid_____
Date _____   Paid to _____   Amount paid_____
Date _____   Paid to _____   Amount paid_____
Date _____   Paid to _____   Amount paid_____
Date _____   Paid to _____   Amount paid_____
Date _____   Paid to _____   Amount paid_____
Date _____   Paid to _____   Amount paid_____
Date _____   Paid to _____   Amount paid_____

DATE _____   **TOTAL $** _____

7b   ANNUAL DEDUCTIBLE

The amount you pay out of pocket before you reach your deductible and your insurance kicks in.

Date _____ Provider _____ Service _____ Amount paid _____

Date _____ Provider _____ Service _____ Amount paid _____

Date _____ Provider _____ Service _____ Amount paid _____

Date _____ Provider _____ Service _____ Amount paid _____

Date _____ Provider _____ Service _____ Amount paid _____

Date _____ Provider _____ Service _____ Amount paid _____

Date _____ Provider _____ Service _____ Amount paid _____

Date _____ Provider _____ Service _____ Amount paid _____

Date _____ Provider _____ Service _____ Amount paid _____

Date _____ Provider _____ Service _____ Amount paid _____

Date _____ Provider _____ Service _____ Amount paid _____

Date _____ Provider _____ Service _____ Amount paid _____

Date _____ Provider _____ Service _____ Amount paid _____

Date _____ Provider _____ Service _____ Amount paid _____

Date _____ Provider _____ Service _____ Amount paid _____

Date _____ Provider _____ Service _____ Amount paid _____

Date _____ Provider _____ Service _____ Amount paid _____

Date _____ Provider _____ Service _____ Amount paid _____

Date _____ Provider _____ Service _____ Amount paid _____

DATE_____ **TOTAL $**_____

7c INSURANCE CO-PAYMENT Usually 20% or a Set Fee
(The percentage you pay)

Date _____ Provider _____ Service _____ Amount paid _____
Date _____ Provider _____ Service _____ Amount paid _____
Date _____ Provider _____ Service _____ Amount paid _____
Date _____ Provider _____ Service _____ Amount paid _____
Date _____ Provider _____ Service _____ Amount paid _____
Date _____ Provider _____ Service _____ Amount paid _____
Date _____ Provider _____ Service _____ Amount paid _____
Date _____ Provider _____ Service _____ Amount paid _____
Date _____ Provider _____ Service _____ Amount paid _____
Date _____ Provider _____ Service _____ Amount paid _____
Date _____ Provider _____ Service _____ Amount paid _____
Date _____ Provider _____ Service _____ Amount paid _____
Date _____ Provider _____ Service _____ Amount paid _____
Date _____ Provider _____ Service _____ Amount paid _____
Date _____ Provider _____ Service _____ Amount paid _____
Date _____ Provider _____ Service _____ Amount paid _____
Date _____ Provider _____ Service _____ Amount paid _____
Date _____ Provider _____ Service _____ Amount paid _____
Date _____ Provider _____ Service _____ Amount paid _____
Date _____ Provider _____ Service _____ Amount paid _____
Date _____ Provider _____ Service _____ Amount paid _____
Date _____ Provider _____ Service _____ Amount paid _____
Date _____ Provider _____ Service _____ Amount paid _____
Date _____ Provider _____ Service _____ Amount paid _____
Date _____ Provider _____ Service _____ Amount paid _____
Date _____ Provider _____ Service _____ Amount paid _____
Date _____ Provider _____ Service _____ Amount paid _____
Date _____ Provider _____ Service _____ Amount paid _____
Date _____ Provider _____ Service _____ Amount paid _____
Date _____ Provider _____ Service _____ Amount paid _____
Date _____ Provider _____ Service _____ Amount paid _____
Date _____ Provider _____ Service _____ Amount paid _____
Date _____ Provider _____ Service _____ Amount paid _____
Date _____ Provider _____ Service _____ Amount paid _____
Date _____ Provider _____ Service _____ Amount paid _____
Date _____ Provider _____ Service _____ Amount paid _____
Date _____ Provider _____ Service _____ Amount paid _____

DATE_____ TOTAL $_____

7d   PRESCRIPTION COSTS

Date _____ Doctor _____ RX _____ For_____ Amount paid _____

Date _____ Doctor _____ RX _____ For_____ Amount paid _____

Date _____ Doctor _____ RX _____ For_____ Amount paid _____

Date _____ Doctor _____ RX _____ For_____ Amount paid _____

Date _____ Doctor _____ RX _____ For_____ Amount paid _____

Date _____ Doctor _____ RX _____ For_____ Amount paid _____

Date _____ Doctor _____ RX _____ For_____ Amount paid _____

Date _____ Doctor _____ RX _____ For_____ Amount paid _____

Date _____ Doctor _____ RX _____ For_____ Amount paid _____

Date _____ Doctor _____ RX _____ For_____ Amount paid _____

Date _____ Doctor _____ RX _____ For_____ Amount paid _____

Date _____ Doctor _____ RX _____ For_____ Amount paid _____

Date _____ Doctor _____ RX _____ For_____ Amount paid _____

Date _____ Doctor _____ RX _____ For_____ Amount paid _____

Date _____ Doctor _____ RX _____ For_____ Amount paid _____

Date _____ Doctor _____ RX _____ For_____ Amount paid _____

Date _____ Doctor _____ RX _____ For_____ Amount paid _____

Date _____ Doctor _____ RX _____ For_____ Amount paid _____

Date _____ Doctor _____ RX _____ For_____ Amount paid _____

Date _____ Doctor _____ RX _____ For_____ Amount paid _____

DATE _____ **TOTAL** **$**___

Monthly Totals for a Year — include Food, Gas, Tolls, Hotels, Airline Receipts, etc.

YEAR   _____

January   _____

February   _____

March   _____

April   _____

May   _____

June   _____

July   _____

August   _____

September   _____

October   _____

November   _____

December   _____

TOTAL   _____   **DATE**   _____

7f   CO-PAYMENT MAXIMUM

Once your co-payments exceed a specified amount, your insurance company will most likely pay 100% rather than just 80% of the cost. Learn what this "maximum" amount is and keep track, so that the insurance company picks up 100% of the costs once you have reached the maximum amount.

ANNUAL MAXIMUM AMOUNT _____

7a Medical Insurance Premium Payments $ _____

7b Annual Deductible $ _____

7c Insurance Co-Payments $ _____

7d Prescription Costs $ _____

7e Medical Travel Expenses $ _____

Other Costs $ _____

DATE _____   **TOTAL $** _____

Note: After your TOTAL outlay reaches the annual maximum stated by your insurance company, they will most likely pay 100% of your health care costs and you will no longer be required to make co-payments.

7g   REIMBURSEMENTS

Make note of all monies you receive from your insurance provider. These reimbursements must be deducted from your yearly medical expenses on your income tax reports.

Date	Insurance Company	Reimbursement
_____	_____	$ _____
_____	_____	$ _____
_____	_____	$ _____
_____	_____	$ _____
_____	_____	$ _____
_____	_____	$ _____
_____	_____	$ _____
_____	_____	$ _____
_____	_____	$ _____
_____	_____	$ _____
_____	_____	$ _____
_____	_____	$ _____
_____	_____	$ _____
_____	_____	$ _____
_____	_____	$ _____
_____	_____	$ _____
_____	_____	$ _____
_____	_____	$ _____
_____	_____	$ _____
_____	_____	$ _____
_____	_____	$ _____
_____	_____	$ _____
_____	_____	$ _____
_____	_____	$ _____
_____	_____	$ _____
_____	_____	$ _____
_____	_____	$ _____
_____	_____	$ _____
_____	_____	$ _____
_____	_____	$ _____
_____	_____	$ _____
_____	_____	$ _____
_____	_____	$ _____
_____	_____	$ _____
_____	_____	$ _____
_____	_____	$ _____
_____	_____	$ _____

Total   **$** _____

Year_____

Add Together

7a Total insurance premiums paid   _____
7b Total annual deductible   _____
7c Total co-payments   _____
7d Total prescription costs   _____
7e Total medical travel expenses   _____

Total Costs (7a-7e)   _____
Minus reimbursements (7g)   _____

Total Paid Out-of-pocket for Year   _____   **Line A**

Gross Income for Year _____ **Multiplied by .075 =** _____   **Line B**

Subtract Line B from Line A = Total Amount of Deduction _____

If Line A is greater than Line B, you can deduct the difference on your income tax reports.

Note: Keep all medical receipts in the Financial Holding Pouch at the back of your Red Notebook. If the IRS inquires about your medical costs they will require you to show itemized invoices and proof they were paid. They will want answers to the fact questions—who, what, when, where, how and why.

To make sure the following information gets to the right people in case of an emergency, distribute copies yourself, or give your attorney copies in sealed envelopes and ask him to distribute them in case of an emergency. Update the list on your birthday.

IN CASE OF EMERGENCY NOTIFY: (name, address, phone number, cell phone, email)

_____

Holds Power of Attorney _____

Financial Adviser _____

Attorney _____

Credit Cards: (name, address) _____

_____

_____

_____

Debit Cards: (name, address) _____

_____

_____

_____

Bank Accounts: (name of bank, branch) _____

_____

_____

_____

Life Insurance: _____

_____

_____

_____

Accident & Health Insurance: _____

_____

_____

_____

Broker & Investments: _____

_____

_____

_____

PART 8
LEGAL

Note: Be sure to make copies of all blank charts before using.

What If

You get sick? What if you're in a serious accident? What if you are unconscious? It's important to think about it now, so you are clear about what you want to happen when faced with a serious health crisis. Once you are clear, you can let others know your wishes should you become incapacitated.

It is inevitable that each and every one of us will die—most likely after sustaining a series of increasingly serious illnesses. Again, the time to think about it is now. Everyone involved, family as well as health care professionals, would prefer you'd spell it out for them in advance rather than be left trying to guess.

Make it Legal

Once you become seriously ill, health and medical issues become complicated and very sensitive. Families become stressed and worried by your condition, just as they are asked to make urgent decisions for your immediate medical care. At a time when they are least able to focus on resources and liabilities, they must address financial issues and assume other serious responsibilities.

It's important to make your wishes crystal clear in legal documents. Having your full input and guidance up front will help your family and doctors provide the best care, quickly and confidently. Two typical documents relating to health care are an advance directive and a power of attorney.

ADVANCE DIRECTIVE

An **advance Directive** is sometimes called a Living Will, a Uniform Living Will, an Advance Health Care Directive, or a Directive to Physicians. It is a document that allows you to make known your wishes concerning your health care should you become incapacitated.

An Advance Directive is a legal document that spells out your wishes in detail. It tells exactly what kind of medical care you approve and do not approve. Even though you may be unconscious or unable to speak, the Advance Directive enforces your pre-stated wishes. An Advance Directive is the only way your family and doctors will know for sure what you do and do not want, should you become terminally ill or near death.

The most common inclusions in an Advance Directive are:

If there is no expectation of recovery:

- I do not wish to be kept alive by artificial life support or extraordinary means.
- I do wish to receive drugs for pain even if it hastens my death.
- I authorize a *do not resuscitate order* (DNR) which means that, should I stop breathing or my heart stop beating, do not perform CPR or place me on long-term mechanical life-support equipment.

(I am aware that often, mechanical life-support is used briefly to help someone return to adequate function and would expect my doctors and the holder of my medical power of attorney to handle this situation sensibly.)

Before Writing an Advance Directive

Be specific in your thinking. What would you prefer to happen:

- In case of a serious accident resulting in coma?
- If your heart stopped beating?
- If you were declared brain dead?
- If you were diagnosed with a terminal illness?
- If you stopped breathing and there was no expectation of recovery?

Are there treatments available you would want or not want to have? Talk with your family and your doctors. Ask questions and get information, but be sure to let your family and doctors know what you've learned and, more important, what you've decided.

Remember, your Advance Directive won't be used so long as you are able to make decisions and communicate them directly to your family and doctors. Also, you can change or even revoke your Advance Directive at any time you wish.

POWER OF ATTORNEY

A **Power of Attorney** allows someone else to act on your behalf when you are incapacitaed.

A **General Power of Attorney** fully authorizes someone chosen by you to act in your stead in all legal and financial matters. It is sometimes called a General or Durable Power of Attorney. These are very broad powers that include all activities involving:

• Payment of bills	• Banking	• Exercising stock rights
• Safety deposit boxes	• Contracts	• Transactions re: US securities
• Settlement of claims	• Life insurance	• Disbursement of any and all funds
• Business interests	• Tax returns	• Government related benefits

- Buying, managing, and selling real estate and properties

A **Medical Power of Attorney** allows you to choose someone you trust to act as your Health Care Agent, someone to make medical decisions when you are unable to do so yourself. Your health care agent can not only make decisions on your behalf based on what is written in your Advance Directive, but can also make decisions from conversations in which you have made known your health care preferences. Usually one chooses a spouse or a child for this important responsibility.

The Power of Attorney and the Medical Power of Attorney are often, but not always, given to the same person. Obviously these powers are only given to a highly trusted person and only in the likelihood of extreme disability. Remember you are asking this person to make the difficult decisions required if you are terminally ill.

Your Health Care Agent will make decisions on your behalf only when you are too incapacitated to speak or make decisions yourself. Also bear in mind that any Power of Attorney you give is automatically terminated at the time of your death.

Criteria for Choosing the Appropriate Person to Act on Your Behalf

There are several important factors to consider when designating someone to have your Power of Attorney and Medical Power of Attorney. Remember, this person will have the chief say in the execution of your wishes overall:

- Choose someone you trust completely, someone who knows you best and would respect your wishes—usually a family member or close friend.
- Preferably it should be someone close at hand or immediately accessible.
- Designate someone who will be able to make difficult decisions and carry out your wishes under pressure.
- Make sure you have the approval of the person chosen before you proceed with legal documents naming him or her.
- Be sure to inform the entire family so everyone is clear beforehand about your choice.

Making the Decision/The High Cost of Terminal Health Care

More than 50% of lifetime health costs are typically spent in the last five days of one's life. If you are clear that you do not want prolonged and expensive treatment in what is essentially a hopeless situation, the decision to create an Advance Directive and Power of Attorney will be extremely important to you.

Convinced? O.K., Let's Make it Legal

- Get the appropriate forms for your state.
- Complete the forms.
- Although it is not always necessary, you might wish to have the forms notarized.
- Before making copies, write on each original document where it will be kept.
- Make copies for your doctor/s, health care agent, and family members.
- Keep the originals in a safe place (but not in a safe deposit box unless your Health Care Agent has the key).

PATIENT'S RIGHTS / DO YOU KNOW WHAT THEY ARE?

Better to know before you need to invoke them. Most hospitals and doctors' offices will give you a copy of your rights when asked. Following is a summary of rights which are spelled out in the American Hospital Association's "Patient's Bill of Rights."

You Have the Right

- To be spoken to in words you understand and to ask for a clear re-explanation.
- To know exactly what's wrong with you.
- To read your own medical record and/or to have a copy if you wish.
- To know the benefits and risks of any treatment, or alternative treatment.
- To know the costs involved in treatment or tests.
- To participate fully in all medical decisions.
- To refuse any medical procedure offered.

ADDITIONAL LEGAL DOCUMEMTS

Living Trust

Any property (cash or other assests) can be put into a Living Trust. At your death the living trust assets go directly to your assigned heirs without going through probate court. You can revoke a living trust at any time should you change your mind.

Will

A will dictates how all your assets (aside from those you've placed in a livingn trust) will be disbursed. It might also list guardians for your children or dependents. A will must go through probate court before your stated wishes are carried out.

RESOURCES FOR LEGAL INFORMATION

Information About Legal Forms and/or Models Can be Obtained From:

- Your doctor's office
- Local hospital
- State Health Department
- State offices on aging
- State Bar Association
- Office supply stores

Every state has an approved living-will document that is downloadable and free on the not-for-profit web site: **partnershipforcaring.org**.

Choice in Dying provides forms for specific states (small fee). Call 1-800-989-9455 or write Choice in Dying, 200 Varrick St., New York, NY, 10014

agingwithdignity.org offers a highly regarded combination living will/health-care proxy called the Five Wishes Living Will which is accepted in 35 states. It costs $5 a copy.

http://www.freebusinessforms.com/webforms/ is a terrific web site for many free generic forms including:

	Form 902	General Power of Attorney
	Form 912	Notice of Revocation of Power of Attorney
	Form 909	Living Will (Female)
	Form 910	Living Will (Male)

Give filled in copies of this chart, in sealed envelopes, to the person holding your power of attorney and to your personal attorney—to be opened in the event of your death.

Location of Important Documents		**Name**	
Will	_____	Social Security #	_____
Living Will	_____	Organ Donor Card	_____
Power of Attorney	_____	Driver's License	_____
Insurance Card	_____	Group #	_____
Medicare Number	_____	Medicaid Number	_____
Safety Deposit Box #	_____	Name of Bank	_____
Safety Deposit Key	_____	Second Key	_____
Birth Certificate	_____	Adoption Papers	_____
Marriage Certificate	_____	Divorce/Separation	_____
Citizenship	_____	Passport	_____
Military Records	_____	Bank Records	_____
IRAs/Roths/Keoghs	_____	Stocks/Bonds	_____
Retirement/Pension	_____	Life Insurance	_____
Deeds	_____	Car/Boat Titles	_____
Mortgages	_____	Debts/IOUs	_____
Credit Card #	_____	Credit Card #	_____
Tax Records	_____	Other	_____

In the Event of My Death

Name _____ knows my wishes and will oversee my funeral arrangements.

Phone #_____   Phone # _____

Name _____ is my alternative choice to oversee my funeral arrangements.

Phone #_____   Phone # _____

Contact and/or Notify

Doctor _____   Phone # _____

Funeral Director _____   Phone # _____

Pastor _____   Phone # _____

Executor of my estate _____   Phone # _____

Attorney _____   Phone # _____

Family Members and friends who will call and notify my extended family and friends:

_____   Phone # _____

_____   Phone # _____

_____   Phone # _____

_____   Phone # _____

_____   Phone # _____

_____   Phone # _____

PART 9
SERIOUS and CHRONIC CONDITIONS

9.1 SERIOUS / CHRONIC OVERVIEW

9.2 DIABETES

9.3 ALLERGIES

9.4 CANCER

9.5 HEART DISEASE

Note: Be sure to make copies of all blank charts before using

LOGS FOR SERIOUS & CHRONIC CONDITIONS

The leading causes of death are familiar and frightening to us all. Just hearing the words cancer, stroke, diabetes or heart disease, is terrifying because we all know someone who is suffering from these diseases, or who is in mortal combat with them.

Any serious or chronic condition requires careful monitoring, both by you and your physician.

Use the logs in this section to record information, or as a model to set up your own logs for such serious conditions as:

- heart disease
- mental health crisis
- allergies

- high blood pressure
- diabetes
- kidney disease

- high cholesterol
- cancer
- arthritis

Also monitor ongoing or temporary conditions such as:

- muscle pain
- constipation
- physical therapy

- changes in medication
- sleeplessness
- osteoporosis

- diet restrictions
- psoriasis

Use the formats provided for keeping track of prevention, diagnosis, treatment, resources and long term care.

Note: If you have a serious or chronic condition, or a sudden serious illness, you will need to set up a separate section for it in your Red Notebook.

9.1a   SAMPLE FORMAT FOR BACKGROUND INFORMATION ON A SERIOUS OR CHRONIC CONDITION

Learn everything you can about your condition or illness. Use the following format to organize the information. We've included completed samples for some of the most common chronic and serious conditions, along with some forms we think will be helpful. Use these as models to create the record sheets or logs you need for your own condition.

Sample Format for Any Serious or Chronic Disease
As soon as you get over the initial shock of being diagnosed with a serious or chronic disease, it's important to take a deep breath and start to gather general information so you will be able to monitor your condition and compare it to what usually happens. Ask your doctor where to look on the Internet and what books to read.

Background information for any serious and/or chronic disease includes:

Disease/Condition _____   **Date of Onset** _____

Definition _____
_____

Cause _____
_____

Prevalence _____
_____

Seriousness _____
_____

Warning signs _____
_____

Diagnosis _____
_____

Usual physician, specialist or treatment center _____
_____

Usual treatment _____
_____

Prevention _____
_____

List of charts and logs for tracking _____
_____

Resources _____
_____

9.1b HEALTH AND MEDICAL NOTES FOR SERIOUS OR CHRONIC CONDITION

Disease/Condition _____   **Date of Onset** _____

Make specific notes of any symptoms, diagnosis, medication, treatment and results:

- Significant events to bring to the doctor's attention
- Severe reactions to food, medications, or exercise
- A new prescription or change in medication
- Specific pain or discomfort
- Severity of a symptom
- Unusual reactions, or any changes in reactions or patterns
- Specific advice from your doctor
- Sudden weight loss or gain
- Side effects of medications
- General complaints and symptoms
- Irregularity of periods

Use this log to keep track on a regular basis.

Date	Event	Physician/Facility
Rx	Treatment	Results

_____

_____

_____

_____

_____

_____

_____

_____

_____

_____

_____

_____

_____

_____

_____

_____

_____

_____

_____

_____

_____

_____

_____

_____

Remember a log is sequential and ongoing. It answers the fact
questions—*who, what, when, where, how* and *why*.

The way to begin making difficult decisions about health care is to educate yourself. Early intervention and informed decision making are both hallmarks of dealing successfully with diabetes. As soon as you get over the shock of first being diagnosed, it's important to take a deep breath and begin to gather general information. Ask your doctor where to look on the Internet and what books to read. You will then be able to monitor your condition, and compare it to what usually happens.

Disease/Condition _____*Diabetes*_____   **Date of Onset** _____

Definition
Diabetes is characterized by hyperglycemia or too much glucose (sugar) in the blood.

Cause
After we eat, food is broken down by saliva, chewing and further processed in the intestines. From there blood carries the nutrients to all the body's cells, including the glucose (sugar) component. Glucose is the primary source of fuel for growing and rebuilding cells, but it needs insulin in order to enter the body cells. If no insulin or too little insulin is produced in the pancreas, or if the cells have become resistant to insulin, the cells become starved for energy while sugar builds up in the blood. This rise in blood sugar is called diabetes.

Prevalence
Over 17 million Americans have diabetes. Millions more are unaware they have it, or they have no idea of its terrible effects.

Seriousness
Complications from diabetes become more serious over the years—especially if undetected or untreated. Stroke, coronary heart disease, kidney disease, nerve damage, blindness, impotence, loss of limbs, and early death can result.

Prevention
Proper diet and regular exercise and an overall healthy lifestyle are known to prevent or stave off Type 2 Diabetes. Also, early detection is key, particularly for anyone with a family history of the disease.

Warning Signs
Sudden, unexplained weight loss, frequent urination, excessive thirst, dry mouth, fruity smelling breath (ketosis), increased or excessive hunger, slow healing sores or cuts, blurred vision, fatigue, bladder or vaginal infections, dry, itchy skin and genitals, nausea or upset stomach, circulation problems (tingling and numbness in limbs).

Diagnosis
You have diabetes if your blood sugar level tests more than 126 milligrams per deciliter after an overnight fast. Normal is between 70 and 110 mg/dl.

Usual Physician or Specialist

Diabetes is most often diagnosed and treated by a primary physician. It is also sometimes found during a critical illness. Other professionals involved in diabetes care: diabetes educator to teach blood testing; eye specialist for annual eye exams, dietitian to develop appropriate eating habits; podiatrist to monitor foot care; exercise specialist to help devise a fitness regimen.

Usual Treatment

- Type 2 diabetes is treated in the early stages with weight loss and exercise. In more severe cases of Type 2, medication is prescribed, plus diet and exercise. If Type 2 has been left untreated insulin may be required.
- Type 1 or juvenile diabetes requires great attention: careful monitoring of blood sugar levels several times a day followed by injections of required amounts of insulin.
- Both types are most effectively treated when daily blood sugar levels are taken, recorded and evaluated.

Charts and Logs for Tracking

Self-monitoring is crucial. It keeps you currently informed of blood sugar levels and lets you know how you're doing with your health care plan. It informs any necessary changes in treatment. Use the logs for daily tracking and for quarterly analysis and checkups:
- 9.2a Log of Diabetes Health and Medical Notes
- 9.2b Quarterly Blood Analysis
- 9.2c Daily Weight and Blood Glucose (sugar) Levels
- 1c Office Visits
- 1e Office Visits—Specialists

Resources for diabetes can be found in the back of the book.

Disease/Condition _____Diabetes_____   **Date of Onset** _____

Make specific notes of any symptoms, diagnosis, medication, treatment and results:
- Significant events to bring to the doctor's attention
- Severe reactions to food, medications, or exercise
- A new prescription or change in medication
- Specific pain or discomfort
- Severity of a symptom
- Unusual reactions, or any changes in reactions or patterns
- Specific advice from your doctor
- Sudden weight loss or gain
- Side effects of medications
- General complaints and symptoms
- Irregularity of periods

Date	Event	Physician/Facility
Rx	Treatment	Results

_____

_____

_____

_____

_____

_____

_____

_____

_____

_____

_____

_____

_____

_____

_____

_____

_____

_____

_____

_____

_____

_____

Remember a log is sequential and ongoing.
It answers the fact questions: *who, what, when, where, how and why.*

This list for good diabetes care is suggested by the American Diabetes Association (ADA), www.diabetes.org. Copy and take these charts to your doctor and diabetes educator when you visit them, especially for your regular 3-months checkups.

Name _____

Tests	**Goals/Norms**

HbA1c (every 3 Mos.) _____ less than 7_____

Weight (every visit) _____

Foot Exam (every visit) _____

Blood Pressure (every visit)_____

Blood Lipids (bi-yearly) _____

    Cholesterol_____

    LDL _____ less than 100 _____

    HDL _____

    Triglycerides _____

Microalbuminuria_____

Eye Exam (yearly) _____

Dental Exam (bi-yearly) _____

Flu Shot (late fall) _____

Quarterly Review w/Doctor

Exams, Tests & Procedures _____

Meal Plan _____

Exercise Plan _____

Blood Sugar Testing_____

Low or High Blood Sugar _____

Low or High Blood Pressure—target 120/80 (130/90 if taking meds) _____

Safety Check on Meter _____

Foot Care _____

Preparing/Injecting Insulin _____

Syringe Disposal _____

Sick Day Management_____

Stress Management _____

This list for good diabetes care is suggested by the American Diabetes Association (ADA) www.diabetes.org. Make copies and take these charts to your doctor and diabetes educator when you visit them, especially for your regular 3-months checkups.

Name _____

Test	YourTarget Goal	ADA Recommends	Needs Treatment Change
Fasting	_____	80-120	Under 80 or over 140
1 Hour after meals	_____	Less than 180	Over 180
Pre-Lunch	_____	80-120	Under 80 or over 140
Pre-Supper	_____	80-120	Under 80 or over 140
Bedtime	_____	100-140	Over 160

Date	Weight	Fasting	After Breakfast	After Lunch	After Dinner	Bedtime	Comments

The way to begin making difficult decisions about health care is to educate yourself. Early intervention and informed decision making are both hallmarks of dealing successfully with allergies. After being diagnosed with allergies, begin to gather general information so that you will be able to monitor your condition and compare it to what usually happens. Ask your doctor where to look on the Internet and what books to read.

Disease/Condition _____*Allergies*_____ **Date of Onset** _____

Definition
Allergy is characterized by an abnormal reaction to a usually benign substance. On first being exposed to an allergen, the body's immune system reacts by producing antibodies but with no outward signs that something significant is going on. After that first and subsequent exposures the antibodies release histamines which inflame body tissues. What we physically experience as allergies is the body's strong reaction to the histamines.

Cause
Allergens can be inhaled, ingested or absorbed through the skin. The most common allergens are specific food such as eggs, milk, corn, wine, wheat, and peanuts; pollen, mold, and household dust; animal dander such as that from dogs, cats, or birds; insect bites from spiders or bee stings; and medications either prescribed or over-the-counter. Quite often the allergen is unknown. Whatever the cause, allergies result in conditions which range from mildly irritating to seriously debilitating. Allergies must be taken seriously because of the ongoing threat to a healthy lifestyle.

Prevalence
Everyone is allergic—it's usually just a question of degree. As more and more people are suffering from minor and serious allergies, they lose time from work and are less able to participate in physical activities and social events. Children become very uncomfortable and suffer loss of energy causing them difficulty at school and spoiling their playtime.

Seriousness
Most allergies are annoying, uncomfortable or irritating, The more serious ones often cause loss of sleep and even days off from work if they become severe. Although allergies are not usually dangerous, they can result in anaphylactic shock which is a severe and sometimes fatal reaction to an allergen.

Prevention
Although it can be very difficult, the best way to prevent recurring allergies is to stay away from the cause. Avoid known allergens if you possibly can. If you're allergic to pollen avoid it by taking your walk mid-day rather than morning or evening. When you come home remove all your outer clothing to the laundry basket, take a quick shower and put on fresh clothes.
- Allergic to pet dander? Don't get a pet. If you already have a pet, entrust it to a family member or friend.
- Avoid perfume, chemicals, cigarette smoke and strong cleaners.
- Keep the house clean and dust free. Avoid carpets and heavy curtains and upholstery.

Vacuuming with a filtered system and frequent washing of curtains and bedding help control dust mites.

- Use a dehumidifier to cut down on molds and fungus, especially in summer.
- Breast-fed babies develop fewer allergy symptoms if the mother avoids highly allergic foods. Breast milk is non-allergenic and provides antibodies that help protect the baby from infections as well as future allergies to food.
- A healthy diet, adequate sleep, and regular exercise help ward off stress and infection which trigger allergies.

Warning Signs

The most common allergic reaction is allergic rhinitis (hay fever) caused by airborne allergens. The symptoms are itchy, watery eyes, sneezing, and runny or stuffy nose. Allergic dermatitis occurs when the skin comes into contact with an allergen that most commonly causes a rash. The response to food allergens is varied, ranging from mild to severe. Allergies can also cause even more serious symptoms such as headaches, frequent sinus infections, hives, eczema, asthma, swelling, stomach cramps, vomiting and diarrhea.

Usual Physician or Specialist

People with serious allergies almost always consult an allergy specialist. However, it is very difficult to find the cause of allergies. An allergist commonly uses blood tests to look for antibodies. He also tests for allergies by placing a minute amount of a known common allergen on or under the skin, and observing the reaction. Other tests involve removing a particular food from the diet and later reintroducing it and observing the reaction if any.

Usual Treatment

- Avoidance: Once the allergist perceives what causes your allergies, he can give you specific advice on how to avoid the known allergens. He can also recommend medications or treatments for any unavoidable allergens. In most cases allergies become a chronic condition. Even the best allergist needs all the help he can get and relies heavily on the patient for detailed input. The more the patient is informed, and learns to avoid known allergens, the more success there is in dealing with the problem. The most successful treatment is systematic avoidance of the allergens.
- Anti-histamines and Decongestants: Most allergies are mild and easily treated, usually with anti-histamines which attack histamine, the cause of swelling and itchiness, or with decongestants which reduce swelling in the nasal passages allowing you to breathe more easily. Both are most effective if taken before exposure to a known allergen. Antihistamines and decongestants are available by prescription in stronger doses.
- Steroids: Corticosteroids are also available by prescription. These "steroids" are used for respiratory as well as for skin allergies.
- Allergy Shots: Immunotherapy involves regular injections of a known allergen which cause you to become desensitized to the allergen. This treatment is usually administered over several years time.

Resources for allergies can be found in the back of the book.

9.3a   ALLERGIES / REACTIONS & INCIDENTS LOG

• When it comes to allergies, you are your own best detective. Therefore self-monitoring is crucial.

• Start this log with a history section where you try to remember what has caused reactions in the past.

• Keep track of activities that appear to cause an allergic reaction. Write down every noticeable allergic event. You might find yourself making many entries in one day.

• Monitor them over time. Make comparisons. Try to see patterns.

• Keeping careful notes will help you learn to understand the source of your allergy distress, and help you to begin to avoid the causes.

• Take this log with you when you see your doctor; it will provide invaluable information.

Name _____

| Date | Location | Allergen |
| Reaction | Treatment | Results |

_____

_____

_____

_____

_____

_____

_____

_____

_____

_____

_____

_____

_____

_____

_____

_____

_____

_____

_____

_____

_____

_____

_____

Remember a log is sequential and ongoing. It answers the fact
questions—*who, what, when, where, how* and *why*.

The way to begin making difficult decisions about health care is to educate yourself. Early intervention and informed decision making are both hallmarks of dealing successfully with cancer. As soon as you get over the shock of first being diagnosed with cancer, it's important to take a deep breath and begin to gather general information. Ask your doctor where to look on the Internet and what books to read. You will then be able to monitor your condition, and compare it to what usually happens.

Disease/Condition ___*Cancer*___ **Date of Onset** _____

Definition
The American Cancer Society defines cancer as "a group of diseases characterized by uncontrolled growth and spread of abnormal cells." Cancer develops when a cell over time changes from normal, to abnormal, to a cancer cell. A healthy body functions by constantly making new cells to replace old ones. Cancer occurs when cells divide and multiply abnormally, causing normal cells to malfunction or be crowded out or starved by the new maverick cells. This sabotage of healthy cell renewal prevents the body from functioning properly.

These randomly multiplying cells may form one of three kinds of tumor or growth:
- Benign or non-cancerous tumors which don't spread and are seldom life-threatening.
- Malignant or cancerous tumors which can invade other organs and disrupt their functioning. They can also spread to neighboring healthy tissue or enter the bloodstream through the lymph nodes. When cancer spreads it is called metastasis.
- Pre-cancerous lesions which may not be cancerous but if left untreated may become malignant.

Cause
Cancer results from a combination of factors:
- Heredity (hormones, changes in immune system, genetic traits, etc.)
- Exposure to toxic chemicals in the environment (radiation, viruses, benzene, asbestos, vinyl chloride, arsenic, aflatoxin, plus many more that are thought to cause cancer)
- Life style choices (smoking, poor diet, excessive alcohol, sunbathing, and poor health habits in general)

Prevalence
The prevalence of cancer is appalling and seems to be increasing every day. Cancer currently attacks more than 25% of the population. Since we are all living longer lives, it is predicted that one in two of us will at some point develop cancer. The most common cancers are colorectal, breast, cervical, ovarian, prostate, testicular, uterine and skin.

Seriousness
Cancer is probably the most dreaded disease—and for good reason. Cancer is always and immediately serious. Great care must be taken, and great attention must be paid—by the patient as well as their doctors—if the disease is to be defeated or kept at bay as long as possible.

195

7 Warning signs from the American Cancer Society
Early detection and treatment are crucial to fighting cancer.
- Change in bowel or bladder habits
- Sore throat that doesn't heal
- Unusual bleeding or discharge
- Thickening or lump in the breast or elsewhere
- Indigestion or difficulty swallowing
- Obvious change in a wart or mole
- Nagging cough or hoarseness

Note: Pain is not a warning sign; it is a late symptom.

Diagnosis
Cancers are found through physical examination and imaging techniques. Lab tests show how much the body has been affected. The broad range of tests include:
- X-rays
- Endoscopy
- Lab tests
- Ultrasound
- Radionuclide scanning
- MRI (magnetic resonance imaging)
- CAT scan (computerized tomography)

Although these tests are invaluable, the most reliable way to diagnose cancer is for a *pathologist* to analyze an actual tissue sample, to do a biopsy.

Usual Physician, Specialist or Treatment Center
An *oncologist* is a doctor who specializes in the treatment of cancer. Treatment often takes place in oncology centers in a large hospital, or in hospitals that specialize in cancer.

Usual Treatment
Treatment choice depends on the type of cancer, the stage of development, and the age and general health of the patient. Generally several treatments are used, either alone or in combination.
- Surgery (may be major or minor)
- Radiation therapy (large doses of X rays directed to the tumor)
- Chemotherapy (simply means using medicine; may be benign or difficult to tolerate)
- Hormone therapy
- Biological therapy (immunotherapy)
- Bone marrow transplant

Alternative therapies—acupuncture, yoga, macrobiotics, homeopathy, aromatherapy, massage, etc.—are often sought out by patients in an attempt to either slow down cancer's progress or to lessen the side effects or discomforts of treatment.

Prevention

Even though we cannot control our heredity and perhaps not very much of our external environment, there are specific ways to help reduce the chance of cancer. However, most studies show people do not follow through on a stop-smoking, increased exercise, or weight loss plan, even though they know the risks. The discomforts of lifestyle changes are nothing, however, compared to the suffering and misery caused by such heavy hitters as heart disease, diabetes or cancer.

A Tip from Ben...

Here's the list, just in case you agree with Benjamin Franklin that an ounce of prevention is worth a pound of cure.

- Don't smoke.
- Drink alcohol only in moderation.
- Avoid the sun; cover up or use sun-block. (If you can see the sun, the sun can see you.)
- Healthy diet—high in fiber and 4-5 daily fruits and vegetables
- Good sleep
- Daily exercise
- Avoid environmental risks, especially harmful chemicals.
- Regular checkups and routine screenings
- Self-exams—breast, testicular, skin

List of charts and logs for tracking cancer

Self-monitoring is crucial. It keeps you focused on your health care plan and lets you know how you're doing. It will provide invaluable information when planning any necessary changes in treatment. Use the *Charts 1a-e* and *Charts 9.4a-g* for daily tracking and for periodic analysis and checkups.

Resources for cancer can be found in the back of the book.

Disease/Condition _____*Cancer*_____   **Date of Onset** _____

Make specific notes of any symptoms, diagnosis, medication, treatment and results:

- Significant events to bring to the doctor's attention
- Severe reactions to food, medications, or exercise
- A new prescription or change in medication
- Specific pain or discomfort
- Severity of a symptom
- Specific advice from your doctor
- Sudden weight loss or gain
- Side effects of medications
- General complaints and symptoms
- Irregularity of periods
- Unusual reactions, or any changes in reactions or patterns

Use this log to keep track on a regular basis.

Date	Event	Physician/Facility
Rx	Treatment	Results

_____
_____
_____
_____
_____
_____
_____
_____
_____
_____
_____
_____
_____
_____
_____
_____
_____
_____
_____
_____
_____
_____
_____

Remember a log is sequential and ongoing.
It answers the fact questions: *who, what, when, where, how and why*.

Be Knowledgeable About the Medications You Take

In order to avoid adverse drug reactions always refer to the medical information sheet when you start taking a new drug, herb, over-the-counter preparation, vitamin or supplement. Be in the habit of keeping the peel-off labels, handouts, or package inserts from your pharmacy, all of which contain important information about your medications. Store them in a Holding Pouch at the back of your notebook reserved for Cancer information..

Keep An Eye Out for the Effects of Drugs on One Another

Because cancer almost always involves more than one physician and you will most likely find yourself with prescriptions from each one, it is important to be alert to the possible effect one drug might have on another. At each appointment, take all your medications with you for a quick review by your doctor's assistant. Take them in their original bottles. A zip lock bag makes a good holder. It is also important that you check for yourself every time a new prescription is written, to make sure there are no contra-indications when used with medications you are already taking. (Note: If you always use the same pharmacy and they are reliable, they will help you track your medications and help make sure they're OK together. However, you must always double-check.)

Include All Drugs and Supplements You Have Taken in the Past

Start with whatever you can remember from the past but don't worry if you miss something. The important thing is to try to list as much as you can remember from the immediate past, and make sure to include everything you are currently using or doing.

List Everything

This will be a running list of prescriptions, over-the-counter drugs, herbs, vitamins, supplements, home remedies and treatments prescribed or used to combat the physical and/or emotional discomfort or illnesses of cancer.

Backup for Your Doctor

This log will serve as a backup for your doctor's files and, of course, it will serve as a good way for you to keep track for your own information.

Give Detailed Information, especially about how effective medications or supplements have been, or if you have had an allergic reaction.

9.4b   CANCER MEDICATIONS AND SUPPLEMENTS LOG

Use this log to keep careful track of all medications/supplements.

Date   Medication   Dosage
Physician   Prescribed for   Results/Reactions
If discontinued, give reason

_____
_____
_____
_____
_____
_____
_____
_____
_____
_____
_____
_____
_____
_____
_____
_____
_____
_____
_____
_____
_____
_____
_____
_____
_____
_____
_____
_____
_____
_____
_____
_____

Remember a log is sequential and ongoing.
It answers the fact questions: *who, what, when, where, how and why*.

9.4c BLOOD TESTS RESULTS GRID

This log will allow you to record the results of your regular blood tests all together on one chart. This will allow you to track your progress and make comparisons quickly. These blood tests are particularly significant if you are monitoring a tumor marker.

Name _____

Date	Weight	HGB	WBC	PLT	Tumor Marker	Notes

As you are diagnosed and begin treatment for cancer you will accumulate telephone numbers, and some fax numbers. You may also be assigned a patient ID number for a particular service. You will need these numbers for your own use, but you will also be asked to supply them to doctors' offices, hospitals, and testing facilities, as well as to insurance providers. Keeping these numbers all together will afford you quick and easy access to them

EMERGENCY

Police
Name _____
Address _____
Phone_____   Fax _____   email _____

Ambulance
Name _____
Address _____
Phone_____   Fax _____   email _____

Fire
Name _____
Address _____
Phone_____   Fax _____   email _____

HEALTH PRACTITIONERS

Primary Physician
Name _____
Address _____
Phone_____   Fax _____   email _____

Oncologist
Name _____
Address _____
Phone_____   Fax _____   email _____

Surgeon
Name _____
Address _____
Phone_____   Fax _____   email _____

Radiation Oncologist
Name_____   Patient ID # _____
Address _____
Phone_____   Fax _____   email _____

Physical Therapist
Name_____   Patient ID # _____
Address _____
Phone_____   Fax _____   email _____

Nurse
Name_____   Patient ID # _____
Address _____
Phone_____   Fax _____   email _____

FACILITIES

Hospital
Name_____   Patient ID # _____
Address _____
Phone_____   Fax _____   email _____

Cancer Center
Name_____   Patient ID # _____
Address _____
Phone_____   Fax _____   email _____

Clinical Trial Center
Name_____   Patient ID # _____
Address _____
Phone_____   Fax _____   email _____

PHARMACIES

Pharmacy
Name_____   Patient ID # _____
Address _____
Phone_____   Fax _____   email _____

Pharmacy
Name_____   Patient ID # _____
Address _____
Phone_____   Fax _____   email _____

SUPPLIES

Pharmacy
Name _____
Address _____
Phone _____ Fax _____ email _____

Health Food Store
Name _____
Address _____
Phone _____ Fax _____ email _____

Medical Equipment
Name _____
Address _____
Phone _____ Fax _____ email _____

HOME CARE

Home Health Care
Name _____
Address _____
Phone _____ Fax _____ email _____

Cancer Support Group
Name _____
Address _____
Phone _____ Fax _____ email _____

Church
Name _____
Address _____
Phone _____ Fax _____ email _____

Hospice
Name _____
Address _____
Phone _____ Fax _____ email _____

Other Support Group
Name _____
Address _____
Phone _____ Fax _____ email _____

INSURANCE

Insurance Company
Name _____

Address _____

Phone _____   Fax _____   email _____

Medicare/Medicaid
Name _____

Address _____

Phone _____   Fax _____   email _____

RESOURCES

Medical Library
Name _____

Address _____

Phone _____   Fax _____   email _____

Library
Name _____

Address _____

Phone _____   Fax _____   email _____

Bookstore
Name _____

Address _____

Phone _____   Fax _____   email _____

OTHER
Name _____

Address _____

Phone _____   Fax _____   email _____

Name _____

Address _____

Phone _____   Fax _____   email _____

Name _____

Address _____

Phone _____   Fax _____   email _____

The way to begin making difficult decisions about health care is to educate yourself. Early intervention and informed decision making are both hallmarks of dealing successfully with heart disease. As soon as you get over the shock of first being diagnosed with heart disease, it's important to take a deep breath and begin to gather general information. Ask your doctor where to look on the Internet and what books to read. You will then be able to monitor your condition, and compare it to what usually happens.

Disease/Condition _____*Coronary Heart Disease*_____   **Date of Onset** _____

Definition
The body is made of cells. The circulatory system is made up of the *heart* which pumps blood, and the *arteries* and *veins* which carry blood to and from the body's cells. A constant blood supply is necessary to nourish the cells and to develop healthy replacement cells. It is a very strong and competent system. However, when something goes wrong we must take it very seriously, because it lies at the very *heart* of our health; it is our *life's blood*.

Some of the major components and concepts of heart disease are:
- Heart attack (myocardial infarction)—caused by a severe blockage to an artery carrying blood to the heart muscle
- Stroke—brain attack caused by a severe blockage to an artery carrying blood to the brain
- Aneurism—a ballooning out and subsequent weakening of the artery wall

Cause
- Plaque—a buildup of fatty deposits which attach to the inside of arteries and impede or stop the flow of blood.
- High blood pressure
- High cholesterol

Prevalence and Seriousness
Heart disease is the major cause of death in America with over a million deaths a year. Heart attacks usually occur in men as much as a decade earlier than women, but 50,000 more women than men die of heart disease each year. The death rate from heart disease is almost double that of cancer.

Warning Signs of a Heart Attack
- Angina or chest pain indicates a blockage in an artery carrying blood to the heart muscle. It usually occurs after physical exertion or excitement. If angina lasts more than 15 minutes it may be an actual heart attack.
- Angina symptoms—a feeling of constant pressure, fullness, squeezing, or pain in the chest that lasts for more than a few minutes or goes away and then comes back. Angina is also characterized by pain in the center or left side of the chest, radiating up, out and down and by pain in the throat, jaw or down an arm.
- Difficulty Breathing
- Dizziness, fainting, sweating, nausea, unusual shortness of breath, or weakness with chest discomfort during exercise

- Indigestion that continues even with antacids
- Not all of these warning signs are present with every heart attack but be sure to get help immediately if it crosses your mind that a heart attack might be happening. Better to be wrong than right and not be around to say I told you so.
- Call 911, don't drive to the hospital. An ambulance will bring oxygen and other possibly life saving treatments.
- Although most men report chest pain during a heart attack, roughly two-thirds of the women suffering heart attacks report no chest pain at all. Women do describe having had unusual fatigue, shortness of breath and trouble sleeping for a month or so before the attack.
- There is also an important heredity factor in heart disease, with children of parents with heart disease being at greater risk, especially if a parent had a heart attack earlier than usual—before age 55 for men and age 65 for women.

Diagnosis

Doctors use several tests to diagnose heart disease:

- **EKG** (electrocardiogram) given routinely to patients to find evidence of suspected heart disease
- **Angiography** uses X-ray to trace dye injected into the heart to check blood flow to the heart muscle and locate any blockages
- **Cardiac Catheterization**—A plastic tube is threaded into the heart, dye is injected, and the blood flow is checked. If a significant blockage is found, a stent (wire mesh tube that holds the artery open) can be implanted, or open heart surgery may be done.
- **CAT** (computerized axial tomography) or **MRI** (magnetic resonance imaging) scans are non-invasive ways to show the heart in three dimension.

Usual Physician, Specialist or Treatment Center

You primary physician and cardiologist (heart specialist) will take the lead in treating and monitoring your heart disease.

Usual Treatment

Medications Are Given for Prevention and Treatment of Heart Disease. For example (because there are many others):

- Vasodilators like nitroglycerin relax the arteries and increase blood flow.
- Thrombolytic drugs break up blood clots.
- ACE inhibitors lower blood pressure and strengthen the pumping action of the heart.
- Calcium channel blockers help open blood vessels and encourage blood flow.
- Beta blockers lower blood pressure.
- Aspirin helps thin blood and prevent blood clots.
- Diuretics lower blood pressure.
- Digitalis strengthens the heartbeat and reduces the size of an enlarged heart.

Surgery is Done to Open a Clogged Artery, Bypass a Clogged Artery, or Replace a Clogged Artery.

- Angioplasty involves using a catheter with a balloon at the tip which is inflated to push aside the blockage.
- Bypass surgery involves using a graft taken from the leg or thigh and the blockage is simply bypassed.

• Stent (open mesh tube) insertion involves using the balloon to put the stent in place to first push the blockage away and then remain in place to prop open the artery.

Prevention
- Stop smoking
- Control blood pressure
- Reduce stress with relaxation techniques
- Seek a doctor's help for depression. (Depression is a big risk factor for poor outcome in cardiac illness.)
- Regular exercise
- Moderate drinking
- Daily baby aspirin (if doctor advises)
- Regularly monitor cholesterol
- Work towards your ideal weight
- Control diabetes

Resources for heart disease can be found in the back of the book.

Disease/Condition   _Heart Disease_   **Date of Onset** _____

Make specific notes of any symptoms, diagnosis, medication, treatment and results:
- Significant events to bring to the doctor's attention
- Severe reactions to food, medications, or exercise
- A new prescription or change in medication
- Specific pain or discomfort
- Severity of a symptom
- Unusual reactions, or any changes in reactions or patterns
- Specific advice from your doctor
- Sudden weight loss or gain
- Side effects of medications
- General complaints and symptoms
- Irregularity of periods

Use this log to keep track on a regular basis.

Date	Event	Physician/Facility
Rx	Treatment	Results / Follow-Up

_____
_____
_____
_____
_____
_____
_____
_____
_____
_____
_____
_____
_____
_____
_____
_____
_____
_____
_____
_____
_____
_____
_____
_____

Remember a log is sequential and ongoing. It answers the fact
questions—*who, what, when, where, how* and *why*.

Be Knowledgeable About the Medications You Take

In order to avoid adverse drug reactions always refer to the medical information sheet when you start taking a new drug, herb, over-the-counter preparation, vitamin or supplement. Be in the habit of keeping the peel-off labels, handouts, or package inserts from your pharmacy, all of which contain important information about your medications. Store them in a Holding Pouch at the back of your notebook reserved for Heart Disease information..

Keep An Eye Out for the Effects of Drugs on One Another

Because heart disease almost always involves more than one physician and you will most likely find yourself with prescriptions from each one, it is important to be alert to the possible effect one drug might have on another. At each appointment, take all your medications with you for a quick review by your doctor's assistant. Take them in their original bottles. A zip lock bag makes a good holder. It is also important that you check for yourself every time a new prescription is written, to make sure there are no contra-indications when used with medications you are already taking. (Note: If you always use the same pharmacy and they are reliable, they will help you track your medications and help make sure they're OK together. However, you must always double-check.)

Include All Drugs and Supplements You Have Taken in the Past

Start with whatever you can remember from the past but don't worry if you miss something. The important thing is to try to list as much as you can remember from the immediate past, and make sure to include everything you are currently using or doing.

List Everything

Make a running list of prescriptions, over-the-counter drugs, herbs, vitamins, supplements, home remedies, prescribed treatments—list anything used to combat the physical or emotional discomfort of heart disease.

Backup for Your Doctor

This log will serve as a backup for your doctor's files and, of course, it will serve as a good way for you to keep track for your own information.

Give Detailed Information, especially about how effective medications or supplements have been, or if you have had an allergic reaction.

9.5b   HEART DISEASE MEDICATIONS LOG

Name_____

Use this log to keep careful track of all medications/supplements.

Date   Medication   Dosage
Physician   Prescribed for
Results/Rections   If discontinued, give reason

_____
_____
_____
_____
_____
_____
_____
_____
_____
_____
_____
_____
_____
_____
_____
_____
_____
_____
_____
_____
_____
_____
_____
_____
_____
_____
_____
_____
_____
_____
_____
_____

Remember a log is sequential and ongoing. It answers the fact
questions—*who, what, when, where, how* and *why*.

HIGH BLOOD PRESSURE (HYPERTENSION)

BACKGROUND INFORMATION
The way to begin making difficult decisions about health care is to educate yourself. Early intervention and informed decision making are both hallmarks of dealing successfully with hypertension. As soon as you get over the shock of first being diagnosed with hypertension, it's important to take a deep breath and begin to gather general information. Ask your doctor where to look on the Internet, or what books to read. You will then be able to monitor your condition, and compare it to what usually happens.

Disease/Condition *High Blood Pressure (Hypertension)* **Date of Onset**_____

Definition
High blood pressure, also known as hypertension, is characterized by constricted blood vessels which cause an increase in the pressure of the blood as it flows through and presses against the artery walls. Picture the increase in flow at the water fountain when a prankster partially covers the spigot and gives you a good soaking. The prankster who constricts the blood vessels is a fatty substance named plaque. The pressure buildup strains arteries and the heart has to pump harder to send out adequate blood flow.

Cause
In most cases of high blood pressure, the cause is unknown. In approximately 5% of the cases of hypertension, kidney problems or a congenital heart defect or other problem could be the cause.

Prevalence
Hypertension is called the silent killer because it has no symptoms. It affects over 50 million Americans. About a third of the people who have it don't know it.

Seriousness
High blood pressure puts the heart and blood vessels under great strain because they have to work so much harder to move blood through the body. Ongoing high blood pressure is a significant factor in coronary heart disease and stroke.

Warning signs (*often none!*)
- Headache
- Flushed face
- Nosebleeds
- Fatigue
- Ringing in the ears

- Heart palpitation
- Blurry vision
- Difficulty breathing after exercise
- Frequent need to urinate
- Dizziness

Diagnosis

Blood pressure is measured with a sphygmomanometer or blood pressure cuff. Normal blood pressure is 120 over 80 or lower and high blood pressure is higher than 140 over 90. Since blood pressure usually reads higher under stress or from excitement or strenuous exercise, repeated readings must be taken over time for an accurate diagnosis.

Blood Pressure Guidelines

	Systolic (mm/Hg)	Diastolic (mm/HG)
Optimal	<120	<80
Normal	**120 – 129**	**80 – 84**
High Normal	130 – 139	85 – 89
Stage 1 hypertension	140 – 159	90 – 99
Stage 2 hypertension	160 – 179	100 – 109
Stage 3 hypertension	180 – 209	110 – 119
Stage 4 hypertension	>210	>120

Usual physician

The primary health care provider is usually the one to find and treat high blood pressure.

Usual treatment

Self Care

- Moderate exercise program
- Quit smoking
- Avoid alcohol, salt and caffeine
- Lose excess weight
- Eat a healthy diet including foods high in potassium and calcium, low in sodium

Medications (antihypertensives) — Combinations Are Often Used

- Diuretics
- ACE (angiotensin-converting enzyme) inhibitors
- Calcium channel blockers
- Beta blockers
- Vasodilators

Bio-Feedback has proven to be effective in lowering high blood pressure in some cases. So has weight loss.

Prevention

In most cases the cause of hypertension is unknown but there are suggested preventative measures:

- Avoid overweight.
- Avoid trans-fats (partially hydrogenated vegetable oil) in all foods.
- Use salt in moderation.

Disease/Condition _High Blood Pressure (Hypertension)_   **Date of Onset**_____

Make specific notes of any symptoms, diagnosis, medication, treatment and results:
- Significant events to bring to the doctor's attention
- Severe reactions to food, medications, or exercise
- A new prescription or change in medication
- Specific pain or discomfort
- Severity of a symptom
- Unusual reactions, or any changes in reactions or patterns
- Specific advice from your doctor
- Sudden weight loss or gain
- Side effects of medications
- General complaints and symptoms
- Irregularity of periods

Use this log to keep track on a regular basis.

Date	Event	Physician/Facility
Rx	Treatment	Results/Follow-Up

Remember a log is sequential and ongoing. It answers the fact
questions—_who, what, when, where, how_ and _why._

9.5d   BLOOD PRESSURE RECORD

Name _____

Blood Pressure Guidelines

	Systolic (mm/Hg)	Diastolic (mm/HG)
Optimal	<120	<80
Normal	**120 – 129**	**80 – 84**
High Normal	130 – 139	85 – 89
Stage 1 hypertension	140 – 159	90 – 99
Stage 2 hypertension	160 – 179	100 – 109
Stage 3 hypertension	180 – 209	110 – 119
Stage 4 hypertension	>210	>120

DATE	BP	DATE	BP	DATE	BP

Remember a log is sequential and ongoing. It answers the fact
questions—*who, what, when, where, how* and *why.*

STROKE / BACKGROUND INFORMATION

The way to begin making difficult decisions about health care is to educate yourself. Early intervention and informed decision making are both hallmarks of dealing successfully with stroke. As soon as you get over the shock of first being diagnosed with stroke, it's important to take a deep breath and begin to gather general information. Ask your doctor where to look on the Internet, or what books to read. You will then be able to monitor your condition, and compare it to what usually happens.

Disease/Condition ___*Stroke*___ **Date of Onset** _____

Definition
A stroke is similar to a heart attack that takes place in the brain. It happens when the normal blood supply to the brain is interrupted or shut off.

Cause
There are three kinds of stroke:
- A blood vessel (in the neck or head) carrying blood to the brain becomes blocked by a blood clot, and cannot carry the much needed oxygen-rich blood to the brain's cells. This is called an ischemic stroke.
- An aneurysm (a pouch that fills with blood in a weakened area in the arterial wall) bursts and causes blood to spill out and damage surrounding brain tissue. This is called a hemorrhagic stroke.
- An embolic stroke occurs when plaque or a clot from outside the brain—often the heart—breaks away, and blocks a brain blood vessel.

Prevalence and Seriousness
Stroke is the third leading cause of death and the leading cause of serious disability in America.

Warning Signs and Symptoms of Stroke and TIA—Act quickly to get medical help.
- Sudden severe headaches with no cause
- Unexplained dizziness, unsteadiness, or sudden falls, loss of balance and coordination—especially occurring with other signs
- Sudden weakness or numbness of the face, arm, or legs, or on one or both sides of the body
- Sudden loss of vision; trouble seeing in one or both eyes; double vision
- Sudden confusion, difficulty speaking or understanding speech

Diagnosis

Because brain cells begin to die immediately when there is stroke, it's essential to get immediate emergency care. Patients treated within three hours of an ischemic stroke (with an intravenous drug called t-PA) can have a better chance at recovering more fully as long as they have no contraindications. The diagnosis of stroke is made by a doctor who examines the patient and uses various tests:

- Neurological testing
- Blood tests
- X-rays
- CAT scan
- MRI

These will help determine what kind of stroke and the extent of the damage to the brain. There will likely be additional testing to detect other possible blockages or narrowing of the arteries.

Usual Physician

Emergency personnel are usually the first to address stroke. As soon as possible they will call the primary physician who will coordinate the care provided by specialists and give information to the family.

Usual Treatment

The most crucial and effective treatment is an immediate medical response and diagnosis of the stroke. The patient must be stabilized and an effort made to prevent additional damage to the brain. Later there will be long hospitalizations and extended re-habilitation programs that will continue even after the patient goes home. Clot-busting drugs can sometimes (this happens in 1-10% of strokes now; most do not qualify!) be administered to restore adequate blood flow to the brain and medications given to lower blood pressure. Anticoagulants or blood-thinning drugs also improve blood flow and prevent the formation of blood clots. Surgery may be performed to open blocked passages, or with hemorrhagic stroke, to stop the source of bleeding.

Therapy

Once the initial phase is past, there may be mild or extensive therapy involved, sometimes for many months. Strokes can be mild or devastating. In either case the patient's will is crucial to optimal recovery.

- People with positive personalities are more likely to recover fully from stroke.
- Low impact workouts help repair damaged muscles and increase your range of movement.
- Be attentive to the affected side which will probably be weaker. Keep an affected leg or arm in a normal position. Have people sit on your affected side so that you turn in that direction and keep that side in the picture.
- Talk about your feelings. You've been through a lot. Talking to family, friends, a cleric or a therapist helps.
- Depression frequently follows stroke, but it can be successfully treated. Do not assume "anyone would be depressed in these circumstances." Request a psychiatric referral if your primary doctor doesn't treat the depression.

Risk Factors
- Age
- Smoking
- Race
- History of stroke or TIAs
- Diabetes
- High blood pressure
- Heart disease
- Atrial fibrillation
- High cholesterol

Note: A headache could save your life. If you have parents or grandparents who had strokes at a young age, especially if they were hemorrhagic strokes, watch out for the sudden onset of unusual headaches. An aneurysm is hereditary, and headaches could signal that it's about to burst. Headaches plus a family history of stroke are cause for vigilance. Alertness and immediate surgery could save your life or prevent paralysis.

Prevention
- Exercise regularly
- Lose excess weight
- Eat a healthy, low-salt diet
- Quit smoking
- Control stress
- Take medications, especially those specifically prescribed for high blood pressure.
- Watch out for diabetes, or if you are diabetic keep your glucose levels well under control.

Resources for stroke can be found in the back of the book.

Disease/Condition _____*Stroke*_____   **Date of Onset** _____

Make specific notes of any diagnosis, medication, therapy and results:
- Significant events to bring to the doctor's attention
- Severe reactions to food, medications, or exercise
- A new prescription or change in medication
- Specific pain or discomfort
- Severity of a symptom
- Unusual reactions, or any changes in reactions or patterns
- Specific advice from your doctor
- Sudden weight loss or gain
- Side effects of medications
- General complaints and symptoms
- Irregularity of periods

Use this log to keep track on a regular basis.

Date	Event	Physician/Facility
Rx	Treatment	Results/Follow-Up

_____
_____
_____
_____
_____
_____
_____
_____
_____
_____
_____
_____
_____
_____
_____
_____
_____
_____
_____
_____
_____
_____
_____
_____

Remember a log is sequential and ongoing. It answers the fact
questions—*who, what, when, where, how* and *why.*

RESOURCES

BOOKS — OUR TOP PICKS

Medical resource books get better and more numerous each year. This list is only a sampling of what's out there. We typically go to Borders and tote a pile of books to a table. We get a large cup of coffee and spend a few hours just leafing through the pages. What we offer you is our current hit parade of terrific medical resources. We hope this list will inspire you to create your own home medical library. Pay attention to your first reaction to a book. You're more likely to use it if it catches your fancy.

GENERAL HEALTH ISSUES - One Picture Is Truly Worth A Thousand Words

The Human Body, edited by Charles Clayman, M.D., DK Publishing, 240 pp.
Another D-K masterpiece. "This exciting book uses spectacular medical drawings, plus images derived from new technologies, as an inspiring aid to understanding the anatomy and function of the body and many of its common disorders. Images work together with crystal-clear language to bring key concepts to life…" (*from the dust jacket*)

New Atlas of Human Anatomy, edited by Thomas O. McCracken, MetroBooks, 240 pp.
A stunner of a book, it is based on the National Library of Medicine's *VISIBLE HUMAN PROJECT* which uses the latest computer technology to show every aspect of human anatomy in photographic and electronic (digital) form. These beautiful images are the basis for the realistic and accurate photographs in this book, which also comes with an interactive CD-ROM Sampler.

HOME MEDICAL GUIDES — The Big Books: Every Home Needs at Least One

Complete Home Medical Guide of the American College of Physicians, Editor-in-chief David R. Goldmann, M.D., DK Publishing, 1104 pp.
Clearer than clear, this is another DK masterpiece. Well written with superb and abundant DK-trademark illustrations. Explains how the body works, describes symptoms, explains how diseases occur, and details modern diagnostic tests and treatments. Includes a comprehensive selection of online medical sites. Comes with the CD-Rom, *The Ultimate Human Body*.

Family Medical Guide of the American Medical Association, Medical Editor Charles B. Clayman, M.D., 880pp.
The 162 page Self Diagnosis Symptoms Chart is excellent. If you're feeling just a little or quite a lot off your norm, you will find out quickly what ails you. In explicating conditions, testing, and treatment, the writing is simple and easy to understand, and is further clarified by clear and straightforward illustrations. The color photos are particularly enlightening.

Complete Guide to Symptoms, Illness and Surgery, Berkley, a Member of the Penguin Group (USA) Inc./ Paperback with CD.
A home diagnosis guide that "explains causes and risk factors, preventive techniques and information that will help you take control of your health."

SELF-CARE GUIDES — Two Great Paper Backs You'll Refer to Over and Over

Mayo HEALTHQUEST Guide to Self-Care by Philip T. Hagen, M.D., Editor-in-chief, Mayo Clinic, 245 pp.
A mini guide that uses clear and simple language, and is packed full of solid information. Includes illustrations and lists, and uses color to separate and highlight. Keep this 8"x10" paperback with your bedside reading and you'll find yourself leafing through it regularly. You'll be surprised at how much information you retain.

Healthwise Handbook, Carrie A. Wiss edited by Steven L. Schneider, M.D., Healthwise Publications, 370 pp.
With its charts, drawings, bulleted lists, clear table of contents, this self-care guide is very easy to navigate. The most immediate answers are presented almost before you've managed to formulate the questions.

CHILDREN'S HEALTH

A Sigh of Relief by Martin I. Green, Bantam Books, 264 pp.
This is the very best first-aid handbook available for childhood emergencies. Kids are so quick and unpredictable that your only defense is some basic first-aid knowledge and keeping this oversize paperback handy. You can find the most important information in 2-3 seconds and "read" the pictures just as fast. The next best thing to having grandma living with you.

The New Child Health Encyclopedia of Boston Children's Hospital, edited by Frederick. H. Lovejoy, Jr., M.D. and David Estridge, Delta, 740 pp.
A comprehensive medical guide is a must for protecting children's health and this one is as comprehensive as they get. Boston Children's Hospital is the largest pediatric medical center in the United States. Their guide offers authoritative information about children's health care, including the most recent medical information.

WOMEN'S HEALTH

The Harvard Guide to Women's Health by Karen J. Carlson, M.D., Stephanie A Eisenstat, M.D. and Terra Ziporyn, Ph.D., Harvard University Press, 718 pp.
A comprehensive medical guide whose aim is "to give women the knowledge they need to communicate effectively with their doctor, and to become partners in taking good care of their health." (*from the introduction*) Over 300 major disorders are listed in the alphabetical guide.

The New Our Bodies, Ourselves by The Boston Women's Health Book Collective, A Touchstone Book, 752 pp.
This book is written about women, for women, by women and continues to be a resource that women deeply trust. The authors operate a Women's Health Information Center and can be reached at P.O. Box 192, West Somerville, MA 02144.

The Female Body: An Owner's Manual by Peggy Morgan, Caroline Saucer, Elisabeth Torg and the Editors of *PREVENTION* Magazine Health Books, Rodale Press, 494 pp.
This book talks to women the way they talk to each other, only with lots more detailed and accurate information. It addresses the female body from top to bottom, offering tips and advice about fertility, pregnancy, menopause, nutrition, weight loss, body toning and other issues dear to a woman's heart and health. It tells what can go wrong and what a smart cookie can do to keep it from happening. Women have unique physical aspects, and having authoritative information so accessibly presented is a real gift.

MEN'S HEALTH

The Male Body: An Owner's Manual by K. Winston Caine, Perry Garfinkel and the editors of Men's Health Books, Rodale Press, 405 pp.
Smart and witty, this guide is a real page-turner. It focuses on how to use and maintain your body properly while keeping a lookout for warning signs, and tells you how to troubleshoot problems. The authors say they want guys to not only be free of disease and injury, but to have a body full of energy, a mind full of creativity and wisdom, and a spirit full of adventure and joy. Part 1 deals with an overview of health issues - nutrition, stress, sleep, sex, energy. Part 2 looks at the body in alphabetical order and tells you how to keep each part healthy and strong. Part 3 is a fitness guide with stretches and exercises. We know men who actually own and read this book.

AGING

Healthwise for Life by Molly Mettler, MSW, and Donald W. Kemper, MPH, Healthwise Publications, 431 pp.
For people age 50 and older, this self-care guide starts at the same age as our bewilderment with the subtle changes in our lifestyle – the ones that somehow just happen to coincide with those also very subtle but very much in evidence physical changes. The book articulates those little twinges and slowdowns as well as those bigger aches and pains, and helps us separate what's important from what is un-ignorable but not particularly significant. And it covers clearly and simply all the physical and mental changes we all must make to ensure that our longer life expectancy won't take us too much by surprise.

The New Ourselves, Growing Older by Paula B. Doress-Worters and Diana Laskin Siegal, A Touchstone Book, 531 pp.
For women over forty, this book was published in cooperation with the Boston Women's Health Book Collective, authors of *The New Our Bodies, Ourselves*. The book proposes that as women come to the end of their reproductive lives (menopause) they are only at the midpoint of their productive lives. In these many pages are found the language, the resources, and the support to make the over forty years a bit more golden than rusty.

PRESCRIPTIONS, OVER-THE-COUNTER DRUGS, HERBS, SUPPLEMENTS

The Pill Book, Editor-in-chief Harold M. Silverman, Pharm.D., Bantam Books, 1151 pp.
Covering 1500 of the most prescribed drugs in the United States, this guide includes actual size color photos of prescription pills in alphabetical order. Information includes: type of drug; generic and brand names; what it is normally prescribed for; general information, cautions and warnings, possible side effects, drug interactions, food interactions, usual dosage, over-dosage; special information for use by pregnant or breast feeding women, or by seniors.

The Avery Complete Guide to Medicine by Ian Morton, Ph.D. and Judith Hall, Ph.D., Avery, Penguin Putnam, 955 pp.
A guide to prescription and over-the-counter drugs, herbs and supplements and their interactions. An A-to-Z listing of disorders, a directory of drugs, herbal remedies, and vitamins, minerals and supplements. Comprehensive and detailed.

ALTERNATIVE HEALTH PRACTICES

Get Healthy Now by Gary Null, Seven Stories Press, 1088 pp.
A Comprehensive guide to natural health techniques including vitamins, minerals and herbal remedies, it covers chiropractic, vegetarianism, nutrition, diet, weight loss, exercise, allergies, major diseases, chronic conditions, women's health, and men's health. It also provides a list of alternative health practitioners nationwide.

Alternative Health, The Hamlyn Encyclopedia of, Edited by Nikki Bradford, Hamlyn, 384 pp.
Printed in England, this book is very British throughout. We suggest it to you because it offers one of the clearest and most straightforward descriptions and explanations of alternative medicine we have seen. 32 alternative health practices are described; they range from acupuncture, through chiropractic, homeopathy, massage, shiatsu, tai chi, yoga, etc. And it does include a directory of U.S. resources.

MEDICAL WEB SITES

Medical web sites hold the key to enormous amounts of information, however the sheer volume can be overwhelming. We have sorted through a great many medical web sites and offer you the best we have found. They are straightforward and highly informative and range over every possible medical topic.

The information contained in the web sites we've chosen range from general information to specific medical conditions. Topics covered include, mental health, health insurance, health news, pharmaceutical drugs, aging, fitness, first aid, etc.

Note: Search the Internet to gather information to add to your own knowledge base; do not use the web as a substitute for your physician's advice and care.

Site Reliability

It's important to question any medical web site's reliability and make sure it's a site you can trust. You especially need to know the identity of its sponsor or owner so you can discern whether the real purpose of the site is to publicize or sell medications or products. Special interest groups might also try to promote their own agenda.

Find out first just *who* is providing the information and verify their credentials; use the "About Us" option found on most sites. Determine if the information is credible and if it is based on scientific findings and has been tested thoroughly. Of course, any information gathered on the web must be checked out with your physician to make sure it's useful for your personal health.

Look for the **HON Seal** granted by the Health-on-the-Net foundation to organizations that promise to adhere to specific standards. There is also a web site called **Health Information Check Up** (**www.kp.org/hicheckup**) which judges reliability, and one (**www.quackwatch.com**) which reveals health frauds and myths.

You can make a good first guess about web sites if you know the meaning of the common endings to web addresses:
- .com and .net — for-profit company or business
- .org   — not-for-profit organization
- .gov — government agency
- .edu — educational organization

If you don't have a computer your local library probably has one and the librarian should be willing to help you get started. Good luck surfing the net!

MEDICAL WEB SITES — OUR TOP PICKS

1) www.healthfinder.gov
Healthfinder is a doorway to extensive government and not-for-profit organizations providing reliable health information on topics from A-Z, as well as health news. Sponsored by the U. S. Department of Health and Human services, its topics include wellness and prevention, diseases and conditions, dental health and general health care, as well as alternative health information and self-help groups. Special health topics are organized for age groups, by sex, race and ethnicity, as well as for parents, caregivers, health providers and others. Also included are dictionaries and an encyclopedia. Information is available in Spanish.

2) www.nlm.nih.gov/medlineplus
MEDLINEplus is the web site for the National Library of Medicine, the world's largest medical library. It offers authoritative information from the National Institutes of Health, and other government, non-profit and health-related organizations. It features current health topics; information on conditions, diseases and wellness; a medical encyclopedia; information on generic and brand name drugs; a dictionary of medical terms; directories of healthcare providers giving locations and credentials of doctors, dentists and hospitals; and other resources and news.

3) www.cdc.gov
The U. S. Center for disease Control alerts travelers to any trouble spots and lists required immunizations. It also provides information about threatening diseases and is especially informative about general health topics from A-Z, including bicycle safety, dog bites, food-borne illnesses, Aids and sexually transmitted diseases, and more. There is a terrific "Hoaxes and Rumors" section which debunks myths and corrects misinformation.

4) www.intelihealth.com
The Harvard School of Medicine along with The University of Pennsylvania School of Dental Medicine provides oversight for this popular web site which has an attractive, user-friendly format. It covers diseases and conditions A-Z; maintaining a healthy lifestyle with information on complementary and alternative medicine, fitness, nutrition, weight management and workplace health; particular health issues of babies, children, men, women, seniors and caregivers; and has an extensive resource section which covers tests and procedures, locating physicians and hospitals and health resources and associations. The *Symptom Scout* is a particularly useful interactive tool, and the dental information provided by the University of Pennsylvania School of Dental Medicine is unique. *Intelihealth* provides reliable material and is a popular web site, but it is important to note that as a subsidiary of Aetna it is a for-profit company.

5) www.4women.gov
The National Women's Health Information Center offers this gateway to federal and other women's health information resources. Many of the materials have been developed by the Department of Health and Human Services, and other federal agencies and private sector resources. It also has valuable special-category sections, such as minority health and women with disabilities, as well as men's health materials. This site is specifically for women and is available in Spanish.

6) www.kidshealth.org
The Nemours Foundation, which operates children's hospitals and specialty centers in Florida and Delaware offers this top site for children's health. It contains information aimed at kids, teens, and parents, addressing children and teens health issues, parent issues, sports, food, fitness, staying safe, and sexual health.

7) www.mentalhelp.net
This site lists issues and disorders centers and more than 25 information centers. Topics range from ADHD, through bipolar disorders, eating disorders, child and adolescent development, OCD, marriage, family therapy and more. Note this is a for-profit site. Three other related sites are not-for-profit:
- The National Mental Health Association (http://www.nmha.org)
- American Psychological Association (www.apa.org)
- National Institute of Mental Health (www.nimh.nih.gov)

8) www.nnlm.gov
The National Network of Libraries of Medicine site will give you the location of the medical library closest to you and their librarians can assist you with questions about medical and health Web sites. These Community Health Libraries can help you locate reliable, up-to-date information on a variety of topics such as diseases, medications, wellness and prevention, complementary medicine, stress management, exercise and nutrition.

The stated mission of NNLM is to advance the progress of medicine and improve public health by providing U.S. health professionals with equal access to biomedical information and improve the public's access to information to enable them to make informed decisions about their health. The program is coordinated by the national library of Medicine and carried out through a nationwide network of health science libraries and information centers.

9) www.noah-health.org
NOAH or New York Online Access to Health is New York City Library's award winning site. Their stated mission is to provide high quality, full-text consumer health information that is accurate, timely, relevant and unbiased. They use recognized web-based resources that are reputable and authoritative. NOAH can be accessed in Spanish.

10) www.nih.gov
The National Institutes of Health is comprised of 25 separate institutes and centers covering diseases and conditions from allergies to stroke. The stated mission of the NIH is to uncover new knowledge that will lead to better health for everyone. This site is offered for your general information. It's important to know to what extent our federal government is working to help prevent, detect, diagnose and treat disease and disability, from the rarest genetic disorder to the common cold.

11) www.mediconsult.com
From this site you can access information on chronic conditions such as diabetes, allergies, lupus, arthritis, cancer, heart disease, etc.

12) familyhistory.hhs.gov
" *My Family Health Portrait*," the Surgeon General's Web-based family history tool. For a paper copy, call 888-275-4772.

ADDITIONAL WEB SITES

Aging
www.ncoa.org
National Council on Aging: 202 479-1200

AIDS
www.aids.org
CDC National AIDS Hotline: 800 342-2437
In Spanish: 800 344-7432
For the Deaf: 800 243-7889

Arthritis
arthritis.org
Arthritis Foundation

Children
www.nichd.nih.gov/
Institute of Child Health and Human Development: 800 370-2943

www.1800hithome.com
National Youth Crisis Hotline: 800 448-4663

Dental Care
www.ada.org
American Dental Association

Eye Care
www.aoanet.org
American Optometric Assoc: 314 991-4100

Food and Drug Safety
www.fda.gov
Food and Drug Administration, Office of Consumer Affairs: 888 463-6332

General Child Health Information
www.aap.org
American Academy of Pediatrics: 847 434-4000

Immunizations
www.cdc.gov/nip
General Information—Centers for Disease Control and Prevention: 800 311-3435

www.vaers.org
Vaccine Adverse Event Reporting System: 800 822-7967

Lungs
lungusa.org
American Lung Association

Mental Health
nami.org
National Alliance for the Mentally Ill

Safety
www.cpsc.gov
Consumer Product Safety Commission: 800 638-2772

www.nhtsa.dot.gov
National Highway Traffic Safety Administration Auto Safety Hotline: 888 327-4236

www.safekids.org National SAFEKIDS Campaign: 202 662-0600

KEY FITNESS AND OVERALL HEALTH — BOOKS AND WEB SITES

STRESS MANAGEMENT

Break the Stress Cycle! By Judith Sachs. Adams Media Corporation

Stress Management for Dummies by Allen Elkin, Ph.D. Wiley Publishing, Inc.

Take a Load off Your Heart by Joseph C. Piscatella and Barry A. Franklin, Ph.D., Workman Publishing Co.

Real Simple Magazine at RealSimple.com

EXERCISE AND FITNESS

Get with the Program by Bob Greene, Simon & Schuster. Clear and detailed guide to successfully and gradually getting back in shape, physically and emotionally.

Prime Moves, Low Impact Exercises for the Mature Adult by Diane Edwards Avery. An "it's never too late" approach to gentle and invigorating exercise for older people who have become sedentary in their habits.

K-I-S-S Guide to Fitness by Margaret Hundley Parker, DK Publishers. Well organized, inspiring, well-illustrated guide to toning your body, staying motivated, eating right and achieving your ideal weight.

K-I-S-S Guide to Yoga by Shakta Kaur Khalsa, DK Publishers. Charts and photos provide clear step-by-step techniques that will introduce you to the physical, mental and spiritual well-being, along with greater flexibility, that yoga can bring you.

www.afaa.com
Aerobic and Fitness foundation:

Video: Connie Love: *Ultra Toner Workout, Beginner to Advanced* (800 222-7774)

Order these videos from Collage Video Specialties: 800 433-6769
- *Nike's total Body Conditioning, Start-Up to Intermediate*
- *Kathy Smith's Secrets—Upper or Lower Body, Intermediate*
- *Karl Anderson: Tone It Up, Intermediate*
- *Molly Fox Shape Up! Total Body Workout, Beginner to Intermediate*

WEIGHT MANAGEMENT—Information about Overweight and Obesity and Help with Designing Your Own Healthy Weight Management Plan

The 9 Truths about Weight Loss by Daniel S. Kischenbaum, Ph.D., Owl Books, 256 pp.
A simple but realistic guide to what it really takes if you're ready to give up the fad diets and the hope of a quick fix. Low fat intake (20 grams a day), daily exercise (30 minutes), and keeping track (write it down) are the three basics of Dr. K's no miracles approach which is amazingly consistent with what every perpetual dieter has learned through experience.

Stikky Weight Management, Laurence Holt Books. "Essential stuff that "stikks" in your head—Stikky Weight Management uses a powerful learning method to teach anyone the skill of managing their weight, step-by-step."

Thin for Life Daybook by Anne M. Fletcher, Houghton Mifflin. A 52 weeks diary and tips from "masters" who have lost an average of 64 pounds and kept it off over 10 years on average. Superb resource.

226

The Complete Weight Loss Workook, American Diabetes Associatiion. Not just for diabetics, this is an excellent workbook—clear and informative.

K-I-S-S Guide to Weight Loss by Barbara Ravage, DK. A typically visual Dorling-Kindersly publication packed with solid information.

8 Weeks to Optimum Health by Andrew Weil, M.D., Knopf. Popular TV guru for healthy living and positive thinking. Has touched countless lives for the better.

The Complete Book of Food Counts by Corinne T. Netzer, Dell. "Contains essential food data (calories, protein, carbohydrates, fat, cholesterol, sodium, ad fiber) for basic generic foods, brand name foods, and restaurant chains." Using this reference you will know rather than just guess at what you're eating.

Adkins Diet Book An alternative to the one-size-fits-all hypothesis of low-fat, low-calorie weight loss programs.

WIN—The Weight-Control Information Network—is the Federal Government's lead agency responsible for biomedical research on nutrition and obesity.
1 WIN WAY, Bethesda, MD 20892-3665
Phone: 202 828-1025, Toll-free number: 877 946-4627
www.niddk.nih.gov/health/nutrit/nutrit.htm

American Obesity Association
1250 24th Street, NW, Suite 300, Washington, DC 20037: 800 986-2373
www.obesity.org is a comprehensive web site on obesity and overweight.

National Weight Control Registry—More than 3,000 people, 18 years of age and older, have lost more than 30 lbs. and kept it off for more than a year, or longer. The average is 60 pound lost for more than 5 years. Half the participants used outside resources to get motivated and keep motivated; half lost the weight using their own plans. www.nutrikey.com/NWCR.html

WeightWatchers.com offers all web site visitors 24-hour access to original articles, recipes, success stories, community message boards and recipe swaps and special features like a body mass index (BMI) calculator.

eatright.org
American Dietetic Association:

ADDICTIONS

Smoking
7 Steps to a Smoke-Free Life. John Wiley & Sons. Uses the Freedom from Smoking program of the American Lung Association to lead smokers through the most highly regarded smoking cessation program.

Substance Abuse
samhsa.gov
Substance Abuse and Mental Health Services Administration: 301 443-4795

SERIOUS AND CHRONIC CONDITIONS—BOOKS AND WEB SITES

ALLERGIES

Allergy & Asthma Relief: Featuring the Breathe Easy Plan: Seven Steps to Allergen Resistance by William E. Berger, M.D. and Debra L. Gordon, Readers Digest Association.
A practical guide giving "strategies for purging allergens from home and office, the best nutrients for allergen and asthma resistance, a review of medicines and suggested breathing, exercise, and stress-relief methods for allergy and asthma sufferers."

www.niaid.nih.gov
The National Institute of Allergy and Infectious Diseases "provides information on the latest allergy research, clinical trials and news briefs."

AAAAI.org
The American Academy of Allergy, Asthma, and Immunology publishes informational newsletters, pamphlets and booklets. It's Web site is filled with asthma news.

Pollen.com
Provides up-to-the-minute pollen forecasts and identifies the levels of pollen in your area and the biggest offenders, be they ragweed, nettle or chenopods. Also has a glossary and allergy-prevention strategies.

Allergy.mcg.edu
This American College of Asthma, Allergy & Immunology (ACAAI) site "delivers information about indoor and outdoor allergies and answers frequently asked questions. *The Allergist Locator* will help locate a qualified allergist in your area."

CANCER

We all rely on medical researchers and practitioners to find a way to prevent cancer, to give us ways to treat it and to beat it. Those of you who are already suffering from cancer, or are helping someone who is, will find your task somewhat less forbidding the more information you obtain.

The Cancer Patients' Workbook by Joanie Willis, DK Publishers, 224 pp.

Cancer...There's Hope; Fighting Cancer; and *Guide for Cancer Supporter*—Free books from the Cancer hotline: 800 433-0464

Men's Cancers by Pamela J. Haylock, R.N., M.A., HunterHouse, 350 pp.

Women's Cancers by Kerry A. McGinn, R.N., M.N., and Pamela J. Haylock, R.N., M.A., HunterHouse, 492 pp.

www.cancercare.org/patients/talking.htm. Cancer Care provides tips for talking with your doctor—"Doctor, Can We Talk?"
Web Sites
www.cancer.org The American Cancer Society: 800 227-2345
www.nih.gov National Cancer Institute: 800 422-6237
5aday.gov National Cancer Institute's nutrition site

DIABETES

The First Year Type 2 Diabetes: An Essential Guide for the Newly Diagnosed by Gretchen E. Becker

American Diabetes Association, 1701 North Beauregard St., Alexandria, VA 22311
1-800-DIABETES Their web site www.diabetes.org offers extensive information and provides an online version of its Diabetes Forecast magazine.

Get Nutrition Fact Sheets at American Dietetic Association, Consumer Education Team, 216 West Jackson Boulevard, Chicago, IL 60606. (Send self-addressed stamped envelope.) Call 800 877-1600, extension 5000 for other publications or 800 366-1655 for recorded food/nutrition messages.

There is a major assault on diabetes and cardiovascular disease called *Make the Link! Diabetes, Heart Disease and Stroke*. Find out more by calling 800 342-2383 or visit www.diabetes.org/makethelink. There is also a diet and nutrition site www.eatright.org.

www.cdc.gov/diaees/index.htm—Department of Health and Human Services (DHHS) and the Centers for Disease Control (CDC) provide the latest research and educational programs.

www.joslin.harvard.edu—Joslin Diabetes Center, Associated with Harvard Medical School, site offers latest diabetes information.

www.healthfinder.gov—Healthfinder is a doorway to extensive government and not-for-profit organizations providing reliable health information on topics from A-Z, as well as health news. It is sponsored by the U.S. Department of Health and Human Services. Information is available in Spanish.

www.nim.nih.gov/medlineplus—MEDLINEplus is the web site for the National Library of Medicine, the world's largest medical library. It features current health topics; information on conditions, diseases and wellness; a medical encyclopedia; information on generic and brand name drugs; a dictionary of medical terms; and directories of healthcare providers.

www.intelihealth.com—The Harvard School of Medicine along with the University of Pennsylvania School of Dental Medicine provides oversight for this popular web site which covers diseases & conditions A-Z.

HEART DISEASE

Live Longer for Dummies by Walter M. Brotz and Rich Tennant, For Dummies.
"Good, common-sense tips on nutrition, exercise, attitude and behavior that can help enhance and sustain physical and psychological well-being to age 100 and beyond."

americanheart.org
The American Heart Association offers print and on line materials about reducing the risk of cardiovascular disease and stroke.

www.heartcenteronline.com
Information on a heart-healthy lifestyle, from nutrition and diet advice to exercise tips. Animations show the effects of high cholesterol and how the coronary artery system works.

www.amhrt.org
State of the Heart program offers blood pressure screenings and educational information for African-Americans in partnership with the Association of Black Cardiologists.

There is a major assault on diabetes and cardiovascular disease called *Make the Link! Diabetes, Heart Disease and Stroke*. Find out more by calling 800 342-2383 or visit their web site at diabetes.org/makethelink.